Hal Higdon's
HOW TO TRAIN

The Best Programs, Workouts, and Schedules for Runners of All Ages

By Hal Higdon, Senior Writer, **RUNNER'S** WORLD Magazine
and Author of *Run Fast* and *Marathon*

Rodale Press, Inc.
Emmaus, Pennsylvania

Notice

This book is designed to help you make a decision regarding your fitness and exercise program. It is not intended as a substitute for professional fitness and medical advice. As with all exercise programs, you should seek your doctor's approval before you begin.

Cover Designer: Lynn N. Gano
Cover Photographers: Tim Defrisco, Rodale Stock Images (front cover photo); Paul Marshall (back cover photo)
Book Designer: Christopher R. Neyen

Library of Congress Cataloging-in-Publication Data

Higdon, Hal.
   (How to train)
   Hal Higdon's how to train: the best programs, workouts, and schedules for runners of all ages / by Hal Higdon.
     p. cm.
   Includes index.
   ISBN 0–87596–352–8 paperback
   1. Running—Training. 2. Marathon running—Training. 3. Physical fitness. I. Title.
GV1061.5.H537   1997
796.42—dc21   97-14947

Distributed in the book trade by St. Martin's Press
   4 6 8 10 9 7 5 3   paperback

—— OUR PURPOSE ——
"We inspire and enable people to improve their lives and the world around them."

In memory of Fred Wilt, a 1948 and 1952 Olympian, a coach at Purdue University and of individual runners, and an author of articles and books that helped many of us understand how to train. Fred was my coach when I achieved some of my best performances, including my fastest marathon time at Boston in 1964. He, more than any other individual, helped me to understand the sport of running and made this book possible.

CONTENTS

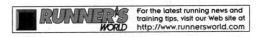

For the latest running news and training tips, visit our Web site at http://www.runnersworld.com

Hal Higdon's Web site, which features his writing and offers additional training schedules, is at http://www.halhigdon.com.

ACKNOWLEDGMENTS

A debt of gratitude is due to all the coaches, scientists, and runners named in this book who worked closely with me in designing the many training schedules that follow. Their innovative ideas made it possible to produce a book richer and more varied than one I might have written using only my own knowledge.

Editor John Reeser worked closely with me in pulling this complicated package together by phone, by fax, by e-mail, and in person on several occasions when I visited him at the Rodale Press offices in Emmaus, Pennsylvania, which is always a pleasure. Pat Corpora, president of the book division, supported us in our efforts. John also was helped in-house by book designer Christopher Neyen and copy editor Jane Sherman. My agent Angela Miller provided her usual direction.

As always, I could not have written this book without the assistance of my wife—and I owe Rose more than the token thanks offered by most authors in their acknowledgments. During much of the period when I was gathering material for this book, we were on a six-month tour of 57 cities to promote my previous book, *Boston: A Century of Running*. It was a hectic time for me, but it was also fun because of her.

Writing *Hal Higdon's How to Train* (my 30th book) helped me to re-evaluate my own approach to competition and fitness. I figure I'm never too old to learn something new that will get me to the finish line a few seconds faster. May everyone who reads this book also benefit from the accumulated wisdom of some of the most knowledgeable experts in the sport of running.

INTRODUCTION

En route to the National Masters Championships in Utah several summers ago, I routed myself through Cincinnati and Minneapolis to save money on the airfare. On the flight from Cincinnati, I claimed a window seat. My wife, Rose, sat next to me in the middle seat. Soon a businessman appeared and took the aisle seat.

Because I was busy working on my laptop computer, I paid the businessman little attention at first. After we took off, I noticed that he pulled out a copy of *Runner's World* and started reading. I smiled and wondered what the businessman would say if he knew that he was sitting one seat away from one of that magazine's senior writers. But he didn't notice me.

I had written an article in that issue about Atlanta's preparations to host the 1996 Olympic Games, but I noticed that the businessman seemed more interested in another article, "The Path to Marathon Success." That was no surprise. Surveys consistently show that training articles are the ones most heavily read by *Runner's World's* readers. I probably write more of those training articles than any of the magazine's other contributors.

The subtitle of the article being read by the businessman boasted, "This 15-week training program will lead you to your best marathon ever." The article included a chart that suggested a series of progressive long runs on Sundays, with hill training or track repeats on Tuesdays and tempo runs on Thursdays. The article was written by Benji Durden, a coach from Boulder, Colorado.

We landed in Minneapolis, and the businessman got off the plane. His place in the aisle seat was taken by a second businessman. We took off for Salt Lake City. I remained occupied with my work; the businessman did the same. Halfway through the flight, he closed his attaché case and began reading the same issue of *Runner's World*. He, too, focused his attention on the training program.

Amused, I wondered if everyone who flew on business read *Runner's World*. The second businessman was not only reading Durden's marathon training article, he was devouring it. Toward the end of the flight, he removed a legal pad from his attaché case and began making notes, apparently plotting his next 15 weeks of training. Surely, here was a man on his way to a new personal record!

We landed in Salt Lake City, and the businessman and I went our separate ways. I ran a 5000-meter race the next morning and spent the next several days mountain biking at Park City. I hoped that the businessman's next marathon was a successful one—but then, we had guaranteed that on the cover of the magazine.

Almost a year from that date, in June 1994, *Runner's World* was on the newsstands (and presumably in the attaché cases of traveling businessmen) with another marathon article. "Run your best marathon with our simple program," the magazine's cover promised. "It's proven. It's got schedules. It will work for you."

This time I had written the article, which included sample 18-week schedules for beginner, intermediate, and advanced runners. The schedules were those that I had helped develop for a training class of runners preparing for the Chicago Marathon. *Runner's World* asked me to write a second marathon training article because Durden's article had resulted in such a positive response from our readers. After continuing reader response, we published yet another training program in the July 1995 issue, also written by me. This one guaranteed to help our readers improve their times and qualify for the 100th anniversary running of the Boston Marathon in April 1996. It featured a training schedule for advanced runners borrowed from Bill Wenmark, a coach with the American Lung Association Running Club in the Twin Cities of Minneapolis and St. Paul.

Programs. Schedules. Charts. Numbers. That seemed to be what our readers wanted in their personal battles for personal records.

Yet as helpful as those schedules were to our readers, I knew there was much more that we could tell them. Prior to the publication of the first article in 1993, I had trained for a spring marathon using a fuller version of Durden's schedule, and I knew that it was much more detailed and comprehensive than the schedule that we presented in the magazine. In the half-dozen pages that *Runner's World* could spare for an article that was headlined on its cover, there never seemed to be enough room to offer as much numbered detail as many of our readers would like. The magazine's executive editor, Amby Burfoot, and I know that, because we receive their follow-up letters wanting to know more, more, more!

Even when I wrote the two training books that preceded this volume, there seemed to be insufficient space to tell all. *Run Fast* (published by Rodale Press in 1992) was subtitled "How to Train for a 5-K or 10-K Race." *Marathon* (published by Rodale in 1993) covered distances longer than 10-K and featured strategies from 50 top coaches. Its subtitle was "The Ultimate Training and Racing Guide." Both books, however, were books of words, not numbers. They taught people everything there was to know about running races from 5-K to the marathon and beyond, but we couldn't devote the space to show them how to train on a day-to-day basis.

This third book completes the loop. It fulfills the promise of *Run Fast* and *Marathon*. Here, we finally have taken the space to offer you those programs, schedules, charts, and numbers. Not only do we provide multiple training programs for the 5-K and the marathon, but we'll tell you how to train, step by step, week by week, for other running distances. There are also programs and schedules for walkers, racewalkers, joggers, triathlon participants, and those returning from injuries. There are programs for high school and college cross-country runners and for youngsters and women.

If you want to improve your strength by doing some weight training, here is a schedule you can follow. And if you want to lose weight, you've purchased the right book.

In the following pages, you will encounter not only programs developed by Benji Durden and myself but also schedules devised by other knowledgeable coaches, including Bob Williams, Roy Benson, and Sam Bell.

The next time I board an airplane headed for Minneapolis, Salt Lake City, or some other running destination, I hope you sit in the same aisle with a copy of this book in your attaché case. I know it will help you in your own quest for fitness and fulfillment.

1

PACE

CREATING A UNIVERSAL CHART

At the end of a class that I teach to prepare runners for The LaSalle Banks Chicago Marathon, I asked if anyone had any questions. One participant raised his hand and waved the training booklet given to the class members. Mentioning the 18-week training schedule outlined in the booklet, he asked, "Could you explain the difference between 'easy' and 'medium'?"

I glanced at Brian Piper, my co-instructor, and we smiled at each other. He and I had visited three of our four class locations so far that week. At each location, somebody had asked the same question, which related to the paces at which they should run specific workouts outlined in the training booklet.

I explained that easy meant a gentle, comfortable pace, one at which you could hold a conversation with a fellow runner without getting out of breath. Medium meant slightly faster, just out of the comfort zone. You could still converse, but not as comfortably. That's a very subtle difference, but it's a very important one for someone who is trying to follow the precise dictates of a training schedule.

Later, as I considered the student's question and my answer, I realized that he had uncovered a flaw in our program. What did we mean in our use of various terms? I realized that Brian and I probably needed to make some revisions, at least in our terminology, before the following year's training class.

Actually, training schedules such as the one used in our marathon class, or those I often offer to the readers of *Runner's World* magazine, are anything but precise. They can't be. Our marathon training class was attended by more than 550 runners. *Runner's World* sells 450,000 issues each month. Individuals attempting to follow any training schedule aimed at the masses have varying degrees of talent and levels of physical fitness. To an elite runner, an easy pace might be a 6:30 mile pace, whereas a novice runner might be incapable of running even a single lap on the track at that pace.

Yet runners want to know how fast to run specific workouts, and it is the intent of this book to provide such information. Let's consider the best way to provide pace information so that you won't be confused if I tell you to run "easy" or "medium."

Developing Pace Sense

There are various ways to measure pace. One is with a stopwatch. Tell a runner to run 400 meters in 90 seconds (a 6:00 mile pace), and it becomes a matter of that runner simply timing himself—or having a coach do it. If he's running on a track, he can glance at his watch as he passes 200 meters. If he passes the 200 mark in 45 seconds, he knows that he's on pace for 90. Too fast or too slow, and he'll need to slow down or speed up to finish the 400 in the planned time—or wait until the next 400 to adjust his pace.

A lot of us who began our running careers as track athletes have well-developed internal clocks that let us know how fast we're running. We developed those clocks while training on the track, usually under the watchful eye of a coach. Runners who don't have track backgrounds, though, need to learn a sense of pace by training either on a track or on measured road courses. It's part of the way we develop as runners.

When a coach works with an individual runner, it's easy to dictate pace. Both the coach and the runner, after working together over a period of time, probably know the level of effort required for that runner to run 400 meters in 90 seconds.

When a mutual understanding between coach and athlete develops, the coach may choose other cues to suggest how to run a specific workout. "Run the quarters all-out," the coach might say, or "at three-quarter speed," which probably doesn't mean precisely that number but some slightly slower pace that both coach and athlete intuitively understand from working together. Consider some terms used by Sam Bell, head coach at Indiana University in Bloomington. In training runners on his track and cross-country teams, Coach Bell uses terms such as gentle, swing, crisp, and hard to tell his runners how fast to do their workouts.

Such terms seem confusing the first time you hear them. I encountered Coach Bell's training terms because I was helping to train a high school runner named Rich Stazinski, of Merrillville, Indiana, during the off-season. After graduating from high school, Stazinski decided to enroll at Indiana University, so I wrote to Coach Bell and asked for a copy of his summer training program. The terms he used intrigued me. He defined his training paces in this manner. (A fifth pace, fartlek, consisted of the four other paces mixed together.)

Bell's Training Paces

PACE TERM	INTENSITY
Gentle	Conversational (not a jog)
Swing	Out of the comfort zone
Crisp	Submaximum effort
Hard	Near-maximum effort

Confused? You have every right to be. The concept is not easy to grasp, although once understood, it becomes simple. Basically, Coach Bell was telling his athletes to run their workouts at varying paces. At that point, Stazinski was capable of running a mile (or 1600 meters—four laps on a track) in 4:30. It took only a few workouts before we figured out how fast he needed to run in order to follow Coach Bell's instructions.

Stazinski's Training Paces

PACE TERM	SPEED
Gentle	7:00 mi.
Swing	6:00 mi.
Crisp	5:30 mi.
Hard	5:00 mi.

These numbers are for a well-conditioned athlete. For someone who is not capable of running that fast for the mile, "hard" might be the miler's "gentle" pace. "Gentle" for many of us means easy walking.

But everything is relative, and each athlete should be flexible enough to define for himself the variables among gentle, swing, crisp, and hard. When Stazinski returned home the summer after his freshman year, he had developed an instinctive grasp of exactly how fast his coach wanted him to run each workout. We rarely used a stopwatch. It wasn't needed.

There's a good reason. Both internal and external factors can change the stopwatch pace that any runner might run in any one workout or over a season. Internally, as a runner improves in fitness, hard might dictate a slightly faster pace, perhaps a 4:45 mile pace. Or if the runner is even slightly out of shape, the pace might be slower. Externally, if the day is hot or humid, crisp and swing might take on different meanings. During the summer, Stazinski worked a construction job that sometimes required him to be on his feet for 8 to 12 hours. When it came time to run in the evening, he had to cope with fatigue, which caused him to modify his workout plan. That's one reason that Bell and other coaches purposely use terms that permit flexibility in defining how fast a runner trains on any specific day.

We want to be vague and offer room for interpretation. Smart coaches realize that training runners is as much an art as a science. Of course, when a runner with a copy of your training schedule in his hand challenges you to define exactly what the difference is between easy and medium—or any other training pace—you owe him more than a vague answer.

Maximum Heart Rates

Seeking to better define training paces for the purpose of this book, I showed Coach Bell's training program to Roy Benson, a coach from Atlanta who serves as a consultant for Polar heart rate monitors. Coach Benson's recipe for coaching runners dictates paces related to their maximum heart rates (MHR). Many runners have begun to train using heart rate monitors, which give them instant feedback as to how fast their hearts are beating.

If you don't have a monitor, you can take your pulse by finding it either on the inside of your wrist or on your throat just under the jawline. Count the beats for 10 seconds and multiply by six. The only problem with this method is that you have to stop to take your pulse, at which point your heart begins to gradually slow down. Heart monitors are more accurate in giving you continuous readings.

The concept of training by monitoring one's heart rate is simple. The harder you run, the faster your heart will beat, pumping more oxygen to your muscles. At some point when running at top speed, however, your heart will beat no faster: You reach your MHR, sometimes referred to as your max. If you know your max, training paces can be defined by percentages of MHR.

There's one caveat that you should be aware of if you plan to use percentage of MHR as a base for your training: Not everyone knows their precise MHR, even though they think they do. One early formula for predicting MHR was to subtract your age from the number 220. A later formula, which was suggested as being more appropriate for well-conditioned people, was to subtract *half* your age from 200. While someone age 40 would have a predicted MHR of 180 using either formula (220 − 40 = 180 and 200 − 20 = 180), different ages result in different numbers. The second formula probably works for a majority of runners, but with my extremely slow heart rate, it doesn't work for me, and it may not work for you, either.

One way to determine MHR is to record your pulse in the last 90 seconds of a short-distance race: 1500 meters on the track or a 5-K or 10-K on the road. This assumes that you have both the physical and psychological ability to go all-out at the end of such a race.

Another way of determining your max is to go to a track and run 800 meters (two laps) as hard as you can, walk or jog one moe lap, then run another flat-out 800. You should hit your MHR at the end of the second 800 meters—assuming you survive, that is. For someone with undiagnosed heart disease, such an attempt could prove fatal. The safest (and most accurate) way to determine MHR is to have a stress test on a treadmill in a doctor's office. Ask the doctor to take you to maximum rather than stop the treadmill early (of course, if problems develop, he should stop the test).

Coach Benson offered some numbers for Coach Bell's paces and suggested names for the different paces based on the training benefits to be gained by running that hard. And because he deals more often with adult runners, who need more rest than athletes good enough to attract college scholarships, he added a pace for rest days that he calls "recovery." (50 to 65 percent). At the other end of the chart, he added another pace that's worth considering: "sprint" (90 to 100 percent).

Benson's Training Paces

Pace Term	% of MHR	Intensity
Recovery	50–65	Very easy (jog)
Gentle	65–75	Endurance building
Swing	75–80	Steady state
Crisp	80–85	Stamina
Hard	85–90	Economy
Sprint	90–100	Speed

We are getting closer to an understanding of how runners of different abilities can define their training paces. But there is at least one more useful number-based way of measuring exercise that we considered before deciding which pace terms to use in this book.

The Borg Scale

In 1959, Dr. Gunnar Borg, an exercise physiologist at the University of Stockholm, developed a set of guidelines by which individuals could describe how hard they trained, from very, very light to very, very hard. He established a numeric chart, settling on a scale that used the numbers 6 through 20. Anyone could use this scale to monitor exercise intensity.

This chart came to be known as the Borg Scale for Perceived Exertion. It provides a function similar to a heart monitor. If your MHR is 200 beats per minute and your heart monitor shows 150, you know that you're functioning at 75 percent of maximum. Using Dr. Borg's scale, you might rate that same level of exercise as a 15, described as hard.

The fact that 15 and 150 are similar numbers is no coincidence. In devising his scale, Dr. Borg pegged it to heart rate. (Add a zero to Dr. Borg's numbers and, if your MHR is near 200, you can relate his numbers to heart rate.) If you use the Borg Scale to monitor your heart rate, you obtain what might be described as intellectual feedback versus the electronic feedback offered by a heart monitor.

Among exercise physiologists, the Borg Scale has become one of the standards for measuring stress. Runners without access to expensive machinery or heart monitors can use Dr. Borg's simple chart to follow the oft-quoted words of advice, "Listen to your body." And the Borg Scale works well. William P. Morgan, Ed.D., director of the University of Wisconsin sports psychology laboratory in Madison, notes that subjects using the Borg Scale can judge their stress levels with great precision. "People are amazingly consistent," he says.

One flaw in Dr. Borg's numbering system, however, is that not everybody has a resting heart rate near 60 or a maximum heart rate of 200. (At the peak of my training, my heart rates were closer to 30 and 160.)

The Borg measurements of stress are worth keeping, but a system that uses the numbers 1 through 10 might be more easily understood by most people.

Borg Scale for Percieved Exertion

RATING	INTENSITY
6 7 8	Very, very light
9 10	Very light
11 12	Fairly light
13 14	Somewhat hard
15 16	Hard
17 18	Very hard
19 20	Very, very hard

Stopwatch times, MHR percentages, numbers on the Borg Scale, and terms used by a coach can all serve to tell a runner how hard or fast to run in a specific workout. By combining all of the above, we've come up with a single, simple chart that everybody using this book can use in their training.

This book contains many charts and training schedules. On most of them you will encounter terms from jog to sprint to define somewhat precisely how fast we suggest that you run. (We decided against a 1-to-10 numerical scale because we felt that using a number for miles and a number for effort in the same schedule might be confusing.) Although we will remind you from time to time exactly what we mean when we recommend running at different paces, mark this page well.

The Universal Pace Chart below is the key to all the training information that follows.

And the next time a student in our class asks Brian Piper or me exactly what we mean by easy or medium, we'll be able to give a more precise answer.

Universal Pace Chart

EFFORT INDEX	PACE TERM	% OF MHR	INTENSITY
0 1	Base	0–50	Very light (little or no exercise)
2 3	Jog	50–65	Fairly light (slow pace)
4 5	Easy	65–75	Somewhat hard (conversational; not a jog)
6	Medium	75–80	Hard (out of the comfort zone)
7	Crisp	80–85	Harder (submaximum effort)
8	Hard	85–90	Very hard (near-maximum effort)
9 10	Sprint	90–100	Very, very hard (full speed)

2

THE LANGUAGE OF RUNNING
A GLOSSARY OF TERMS

Each sport has its terms, which need to be defined for those unfamiliar with the sport and maybe even for those who consider themselves familiar. Running is no different. Someone who is learning how to train to improve performance must come to grips with terms such as *fartlek* and *surges* and will probably need to learn the subtle difference between running repeats and doing interval training.

In two of my previous books, I sometimes devoted pages or entire chapters to defining terms. That won't be entirely necessary for this book, but you will have an easier time understanding the many charts and schedules that follow if you learn the basic terms used by coaches to describe different types of training. Here is a glossary of training terms to help you reach your running goals.

Aerobic. Literally, "with air." This describes running at a pace slow enough that you can converse comfortably with your running partner. Theoretically at least, you should be able to run forever at this pace.

Aerobics. Originally the title of a best-selling book by Kenneth H. Cooper, M.D., president and founder of the Cooper Aerobics Center in Dallas. This groundbreaking book touted the health benefits of exercise. The term *aerobics* now has come to mean various types of exercise (walking, running, swimming, cycling, cross-training) that allow people who exercise to improve their physical fitness.

Age groups. Most races have age groups or classes to recognize the fact that speeds change with age. Children get faster as they get older, but adults usually slow down as they age. Typically, the divisions are in two-year increments for children, which may vary from event to event, and five-year increments for adults: 20 to 24, 25 to 29, 30 to 34, and so on. Classifying runners by age lies at the heart of the masters movement, which has separate competitions for runners over age 40.

Anaerobic. Literally, "without air." When you exercise at a high level, your cardiovascular system can no longer process oxygen fast enough to clear the waste products connected with energy production (mainly lactic acid). This eventually forces you to slow down or stop.

Anaerobic threshold. Abbreviated A.T., as in A.T. training. Also known as lactate threshold, this is the point at which the body (at least theoretically) switches from an aerobic to an anaerobic state. Actually, the two states blend together, but there is a point at which lactic acid begins to accumulate faster than the cardiovascular system can eliminate it. If, by training hard, you can raise your lactate threshold, you should be able to perform at a higher level.

Boston Marathon. The Holy Grail for most endurance runners, this mid-April race sponsored by the Boston Athletic Association is special because you have to qualify for entry by running a fast previous marathon. Men ages 18 to 34 must run 3:10, and women the same age must do 3:40, with graduated standards (5 minutes for every five years) for older runners. The 100th running of the Boston Marathon in 1996 attracted 38,000 entrants and was considered by runners to be the most important running event of the century.

Bounding. A routine to improve speed and flexibility that includes various drills such as skipping, hopping, and running with high knee lifts or high back kicks.

Carbohydrate. Foods contain protein, fat, and carbohydrate. All are necessary for good health, but carbohydrates are the preferred food for athletes because they are easy to digest and convert quickly to energy. Typical carbohydrate-rich foods are potatoes, rice, fruits, breads, cereals, and pasta (one reason that runners often eat spaghetti the night before a marathon). A good nutritional balance is 15 percent proteins, 30 percent fats, and 55 percent carbohydrates.

Carbo-loading. Originally, this term described an extreme pre-race regimen that involved a depletion run of 20 miles one week before a marathon, then three days of a high-fat diet followed by three days of a high-carbohydrate diet. Presumably, this forced the muscles to store more glycogen, the main energy source for fueling muscles. Later, scientists determined that runners could get similar results by skipping the high-fat phase and concentrating mainly on the high-carbohydrate phase. The term today refers to any pre-race diet that is high in carbohydrates.

Cooldown. Usually employed by runners at the end of a speed workout or a race to prevent next-day muscle stiffness, although the main benefit of cooling down may be as much psychological as physical. A cooldown signals the end of the workout much as the warmup signals the beginning. A cooldown usually consists of easy jogging but may contain strides or stretching.

Crisp. A training pace defined as running at 80 to 85 percent of your maximum heart rate, or a submaximum effort. This is the pace at which serious runners improve performance, but you can only train at this pace (or faster) occasionally without increasing your risk of injury.

Cross-training. Any type of sports activity that is different from your main sport yet still increases your physical fitness. For instance, runners often cross-train by swimming, cycling, or lifting weights. Cross-training is good for developing general fitness, but it should be practiced judiciously so you do not develop muscles that are antagonistic to those used in your main sport.

Easy. A training pace defined as running at 65 to 75 percent of your maximum heart rate. It is a conversational level, but somewhat faster than a jog.

Fartlek. Swedish for "speed play." A training method developed in Sweden during the 1940s by Coach Gosta Holmer. Milers Gunnar Haag and Arne Anderson would run in the woods, alternating slow and fast running at varying distances over undulating terrain, training almost instinctively.

Fluid replacement. During exercise, the body cools itself by sweating. Fluids lost by sweating must be replaced to avoid overheating during a workout or race and also to prevent chronic dehydration, which can inhibit training. Water is the preferred (and cheapest) replacement beverage; various commercial electrolyte replacement drinks also provide extra energy.

Glycogen. The main energy source for fueling muscles. Before the body can burn carbohydrate or fat, it must be converted into glycogen. Once glycogen is depleted, the body must rely on fat, a less efficient fuel source, for energy. One reason that runners "hit the wall" at 20 miles during a marathon is that their muscles have become depleted of glycogen.

Hard. A training pace defined as running at 85 to 90 percent of your maximum heart rate, or a near-maximum effort. Most runners probably don't achieve this pace except during short training runs on the track or during races.

Hard/easy. A popular training pattern popularized by former University of Oregon track coach Bill Bowerman. Bowerman believes that in order to run hard one day, you have to run easy the day before (or for some days before). Bowerman's hard/easy pattern of balancing stress with rest is generally accepted as the most effective pattern for improving performance.

Heart monitor. A handy training device that usually consists of a chest strap that holds a monitor to measure heartbeats and transmit the information to a wristwatch. No guessing here: You can determine your exact level of exertion.

Hill training. New Zealand coach Arthur Lydiard popularized this form of training in which runners do repeat, short runs up a hill rather than on a track. One advantage of hill training is that it develops your quadriceps muscles and your ability to lift your legs. Another advantage is that there's less impact on your legs while running up hills. Many experienced runners use hill training during one phase of their training to prepare themselves to move to the track during a later phase.

Interval training. A speed workout that usually features multiple repeat runs in which the rest between repeats is controlled as carefully as the speed of the repeats. An example would be running 10 × 400 meters in 70 seconds and jogging 200 meters in 90 seconds between the repeats. The interval between the repeats gives this type of training its name.

Jog. Slow running. For the purposes of this book, a jog is defined as running at 50 to 65 percent of your maximum heart rate.

Jogger; jogging. Familiar terms used to describe people who run noncompetitively. The late George Sheehan, M.D., a well-known *Runner's World* columnist, once described the difference between a jogger and a runner as an entry blank to a race.

Lactic acid. A by-product of energy production, lactic acid accumulates in the muscles during anaerobic training. At high concentrations, this causes the muscles to perform less efficiently. Despite what some runners believe, lactic acid does *not* cause next-day muscle soreness. Usually, it clears from the system within 20 to 30 minutes after hard, anaerobic training.

Long run. Typically, most distance runners do at least one long run a week of anywhere from 6 to 20 miles. The purpose is to build an endurance base and improve the body's ability to burn fats and preserve glycogen. It's best to do long runs at a speed slower than race pace.

Marathon. The classic long-distance race: 26 miles 385 yards, or 42.2 kilometers. Marathon was the name of the Greek plain where the Athenians defeated an invading army of Persians in 490 B.C. After the battle (according to legend), a warrior-messenger named Pheidippides ran to Athens and died saying, "Rejoice, we conquer!" A "marathon" over the legendary route run by Pheidippides was added to the Olympic Games in 1896. We have been running marathons ever since.

Massage. Massage therapists have become very popular with endurance athletes who are seeking to recover after hard workouts or long races. Little scientific evidence supports the suggestion that massage helps recovery, but it certainly promotes relaxation. The best time for a postrace massage is 24 to 72 hours after the race, when muscle soreness peaks.

Masters. Competitors over the age of 40 are classified as masters. Women, however, compete at age 35 at the World Veterans Championships, and some track meets include submasters competitions for athletes ages 30 to 39. Masters usually compete in five-year age divisions. (Although Americans use the name masters, the preferred international term is *veterans*.) The main publication for masters athletes is *National Masters News*, P.O. Box 50098, Eugene, OR 97401; phone (541) 343-7716.

Max. Short for "maximum." Exercise scientists sometimes use max to describe the maximum volume of oxygen that the cardiovascular system can process during exercise, written as "VO_2 max." When you encounter the term in this book, however, it refers to maximum heart rate.

Maximum heart rate (MHR). As you run faster or longer, your heartbeat will increase to a point where it finally can increase no more. This is your maximum heart rate, a handy tool for measuring how hard you're training. If your max is 200 and your heart is beating at 150 beats a minute, you are said to be training at 75 percent.

Various formulas are used to predict maximum heart rate; the best known is 220 minus your age. Kenneth H. Cooper, M.D., president and founder of the Cooper Aerobics Center in Dallas, however, considers 200 minus half your age a better predictor for people who exercise. But individuals differ, and the only way to accurately determine your maximum heart rate is to take a treadmill stress test.

Medium. A training pace defined as running at 75 to 80 percent of your maximum heart rate, or "out of the comfort zone." You can probably still hold a conversation, but not as easily as while running at an easy pace.

Meters. With the exception of a few English-speaking countries, the world operates on the metric system. Runners probably understand meters better than most Americans, because we run 5-K (5000 meters) and 10-K (10,000 meters) race distances and discover that we have gone a little over 3 or 6 miles. Most tracks are 400 meters long, or close to a quarter-mile. The Olympic distance of 1500 meters is thus about 100 meters less than a mile.

Number placement. Distance runners competing in road races generally pin their numbers to the front of their shirts so they can be identified as they approach. Track athletes generally pin their numbers on their backs so they can be identified after crossing the line. This is a small but significant fact to know if you are competing in your first road race or track meet.

Olympic Games. An athletic competition begun in ancient Greece (the first recorded event was in 776 B.C.), this quadrennial, multi-sports competition was revived by Baron Pierre de Coubertin, a French nobleman, in Athens, Greece, in 1896. The showcase sport of the Olympics is track and field, including the marathon. Most people in the world consider the Olympic Games to be the world's greatest sporting event.

Performance predictions. If you know your times for one race distance, you probably can predict your performance for other distances, including the marathon. One marathon prediction formula involves multiplying your current 10-K best by 4.66. Two books that include extensive prediction charts are *Oxygen Power* (available from Jack Daniels, Ph.D., Box 5062, Cortland, NY 13045) and *Running Trax: Computerized Running Training Programs* by J. Gerry Purdy (available from *Track & Field News*, 2570 El Camino Real, Suite 606, Los Altos, CA 94040).

Quarters. Repeats of 400 meters, run on a track. The term arose when tracks were a quarter-mile long, and it has not changed despite races being run in meters. Similarly, halfs are 800 meters run in training.

Race pace. The pace at which you will run the event for which you are training. If you are planning to run a 3-hour marathon, for example, race pace for you would be about 7:00 per mile. For someone capable of 31:00 for a 10-K, race pace would be 75-second quarters. One reason for training at race pace is that it accustoms the body to running comfortably at the speed used in competition.

Recovery. Recovery is what you do between hard workouts. There's a subtle difference between *recovery* and *rest* as the terms are used by some coaches. A rest day would more likely be one on which you do no training. On a recovery day you might run easy or cross-train.

Repeats. A training distance that is run more than once in a workout. For example, in 3 × 400 meters, the 400 is the repeat, sometimes referred to as a rep, as in repetition. The term is often used in describing speedwork. A repeat workout is one in which repeats are run, usually with relatively long rest periods between repetitions, such as walking between 400s rather than jogging between them as in interval training.

Rest. A sometimes-overlooked component of any successful training plan. Muscles exercised to near exhaustion need time to recover, sometimes 24 to 72 hours. Insufficient rest can result in overtraining, chronic fatigue, and reduced performance.

Speedwork. Any form of training that is done at a faster pace than usual, such as repeats on the track. One benefit of speedwork is that it allows you to accustom your muscles to the stress of running at the pace you will use in races. In this respect, speedwork can provide great training benefits, but running fast too often raises the risk of injury.

Splits. After the notorious Rosie Ruiz was presented with the laurel wreath for "winning" the 1980 Boston Marathon, TV commentator Kathrine Switzer asked Ruiz what her splits were. Ruiz replied, "What are splits?" That confirmed for Switzer that Ruiz was an impostor who had not run the whole distance. Splits are times that are recorded or remembered during a race, usually every mile in marathons or every 400 meters in track races. As it says on the T-shirt, "It's a running thing."

Sprint. At track-and-field meets, races between 100 and 400 meters are considered sprints. The term is also used to describe running full speed. For the purposes of this book, a sprint is defined as running at 90 to 100 percent of your maximum heart rate.

Strength training. Weightlifting and working out by using exercise machines can improve your strength. Whether or not extra strength equals improved performance for distance runners is debatable, but strength training certainly can improve your overall fitness. The two groups most likely to benefit from strength training are women and masters. Unless you have a knowledgeable strength trainer who knows what he is doing, combining low weights and high reps and focusing more on the upper body seems to work best for distance runners.

Stress test. A test to determine cardiovascular fitness, usually done in a laboratory or doctor's office. Most often a treadmill is used for the test, with the runner (or walker) going progressively harder until he can go no further. Doctors give stress tests to diagnose heart disease. Scientists use them for research. A stress test is the best way to determine your maximum heart rate.

You can also determine your maximum heart rate in a field test by using a heart monitor, although some risk is involved with this method (particularly for those with undiagnosed heart problems). Warm up thoroughly, then run 2 × 800 meters at full speed, jogging 400 meters between repeats. Your heart should hit max at the end of the second 800. Or you can check your heartbeat while sprinting toward the finish of a 5-K or 10-K race.

Stretching. A static form of exercise in which you assume a position that stretches one or more muscles, then hold that position for a length of time. Scientists still debate whether or not stretching can help prevent injuries, but it certainly does promote flexibility. The best time to stretch is after you've warmed your muscles. Two important rules: Don't bounce and don't overstretch.

Strides. Sprints of 50 to 150 meters done at a level somewhat below full speed. You might call them slow sprints. They are useful during warmups and cooldowns to prepare the body to run fast or to recover after running fast. A typical stride session might involve four laps on the track, sprinting (or striding) the straightaways.

Surge. This term relates to a sudden increase in pace, either in a race or in training. In a race, a runner suddenly surges to lose or weaken an opponent. In training, a runner surges to increase leg speed as well as to develop the ability to execute this tactic in a race.

Taper. To rest their muscles and ensure peak performance, runners usually cut back their training anywhere from one day to three weeks before a major competition. Knowing how and when to taper is a skill learned through experience.

Tempo run. Also called a lactate threshold run or A.T. (anaerobic threshold) run, this is a type of training popularized by Jack Daniels, Ph.D., cross-country and track-and-field coach at the State University of New York in Cortland. This workout usually involves a run of 30 to 60 minutes that starts easy, builds to a steady speed in the middle, then ends easy. Tempo runs offer a very effective way to build speed endurance without the stress or risk of speedwork.

Training effect. Benefits accrued from exercise. There is a theoretical level (probably 50 to 60 percent of your maximum heart rate) above which the exercise you are doing will improve your physical fitness.

Ultramarathon. Any race longer than the marathon distance of 26 miles 385 yards (42.2 kilometers). Runners often shorten the term and refer to running ultras.

Veterans. The international term used to describe male competitors over the age of 40 or female competitors over the age of 35. The popular American term for runners in these age groups is *masters*.

Warmup. Before a speed workout or a race, runners usually warm up their muscles. A typical warmup might include one to two miles of easy jogging, rest, stretching, strides, and possibly bounding drills, followed by some more easy jogging.

3

BEGINNERS
CHUCK CORNETT'S
35-DAY PROGRAM

Chuck Cornett remembers a real estate broker who joined the fitness class that he teaches in Jacksonville, Florida: "She was 52 years old, 5 feet 2 inches tall, and 217 pounds. Sitting in the classroom, her heart rate was 135 beats per minute. She was already in the 'target training zone,' and she hadn't even gotten off the bench."

Cornett, a retired U.S. Navy pilot who has guided more than 20,000 people in his "Top Run" program for beginning walkers and runners, showed the woman how to train. He told her about his five-week program, which is so simple that it almost defies explanation.

Those in Cornett's program are told to exercise no more than a half-hour a day for 35 days. Here is what they do the first day.

• Stretch briefly.
• Walk out the door in any direction.
• Go for 15 minutes. (Distance doesn't matter.)

- Turn around and return home.
- The first 5 minutes is *easy* walking. (This is mandatory.)
- The last 5 minutes is *easy* walking. (This is also mandatory.)
- During the middle 20 minutes, they are free to walk or jog.

For the following 34 days—a total of five weeks—the beginners do exactly the same workout.

"The only difference," Cornett says, "is that as they begin to feel fit and shed a few pounds, they're motivated and encouraged to walk or jog somewhat faster during the middle 20 minutes of the workouts. But they decide that portion of their workouts. I don't provide them with a day-by-day schedule, which frightens many beginners."

This is Cornett's 35-day program for beginners. With such simple commitments, miracles occur. In the case of the real estate broker, she remained in the program after the initial five weeks and eventually slimmed down to 135 pounds. "She also doubled her income and now has a bunch of guys chasing her," laughs Cornett. The real estate broker also went on to finish a marathon, but Cornett warns, "Running marathons is not necessarily our goal. The main goal is fitness and feeling good about yourself. That's a goal that's much more easily attainable than many out-of-shape people think."

Moderation and Motivation

Cornett knows what it feels like both to be in and out of shape. In high school in Bell City, Louisiana, he ran the mile in 4:44. He enlisted in the U.S. Navy at age 17 and rose through the ranks to become a captain, piloting the multi-engine P-3 Orion, an anti-submarine-warfare craft. But over the period of a quarter-century, he had allowed himself to get sadly out of shape.

"At that time, running was used as punishment in the military," Cornett says. "If you did something wrong, you did double-time with a rifle around the parade grounds. As I grew older, on the few occasions I tried running, it was too fast, too hard, too painful."

In 1978, Cornett was 44 years old and weighed 196 pounds, 63 pounds more than he had as a high school athlete. He smoked three packs of cigarettes a day while living in Orlando and serving as commander of Florida's Naval Recruiting District. "I woke up one morning feeling so rotten that I thought I was having a heart attack," he recalls. "A physical exam proved that was not the case, but it caused me to look in the mirror and re-evaluate my lifestyle."

Cornett designed a 35-day program for getting into shape. "The program had one participant: me." He started walking and jogging, changed his diet, and stopped smoking. He noticed a remarkable change in stress levels and an increase in energy. After he retired from the Navy in 1980, he began showing others how they could modify their lifestyles.

He believes in moderation. His motto is "No pain, high gain." He defines his usual clientele as being 6-F: "...in their forties or fifties, fat, flabby, fed-up, and wanting to fix it." He also works with people in retirement centers. Cornett describes one center where the people in his class averaged 76 years of age: "The youngest was 67; the oldest was a woman of 92 who had had three strokes. At the end of five weeks, we had doubled her strength and the distance she could walk during the exercise period."

He also believes in motivation, saying, "It is important for beginners to exercise every day for the first 35 days in order to make it a habit. After 35 days, I have them hooked. If they walk briskly, they'll be covering 1.5 to 2 miles during the half-hour period. In a week, they'll go 10 to 14 miles. That's close to the weekly mileage that Kenneth H. Cooper, M.D., president and founder of the Cooper Aerobics Center in Dallas, says is needed for fitness."

Maintaining Fitness

After five weeks, the people in Cornett's classes move to the next level of fitness. They are no longer beginners; they are exercisers or fitness walkers, and some may proceed to become racers or even marathoners. Cornett, however, emphasizes that the goal of his program is *not* to teach people how to compete. "If they want to use races as goals, I'll help," he says, "but I'm happy simply to show formerly sedentary people how to maintain a base level of fitness for the rest of their lives."

Thirty minutes a day of almost any exercise can do just that, but Cornett finds that people in his program want somewhat more structure for both maintaining and increasing base fitness. For them, he offers a step upward that focuses less on minutes and more on miles. In the next five weeks, Cornett's beginners train by walking or jogging the mileages shown in the table below.

Weeks 6 through 10

WEEK	MON.	TUES.	WED.	THURS.	FRI.	SAT.	SUN.	WEEKLY MILEAGE
6	Rest	3 mi. easy or medium	2 mi. easy	3 mi. easy or medium	2 mi. easy	Rest	5 mi. easy or medium	15
7	Rest	3 mi. easy or medium	2 mi. easy	4 mi. easy or medium	2 mi. easy	Rest	5 mi. easy or medium	16
8	1 mi. easy	3 mi. easy or medium	2 mi. easy	4 mi. easy or medium	2 mi. easy	Rest	5 mi. easy or medium	17
9	2 mi. easy	3 mi. easy or medium	2 mi. easy	4 mi. easy or medium	2 mi. easy	Rest	6 mi. easy or medium	19
10	Rest	2 mi. easy or medium	1 mi. easy	2 mi. easy or medium	1 mi. easy	Rest	4 mi. easy or medium	10

As the beginning exercisers in his program progress and become more fit, Cornett continues to increase their levels of training. At this point he also adds rest days, usually before and/or after the days on which participants run their longest and hardest workouts. For the next five weeks (35 more days), Cornett's beginners train according to the schedule on page 24.

After 10 weeks (a total of 70 days), Cornett feels that his beginners have achieved a level of fitness that they can maintain forever. He has them continue to train at the same level shown in weeks 8 and 9 above, using the final week as a rest week. They can continue to train at this maintenance level indefinitely, modifying the program to fit their own needs from week to week and month to month. The table below shows how Cornett's beginners maintain fitness.

Weeks 11 through 15

WEEK	MON.	TUES.	WED.	THURS.	FRI.	SAT.	SUN.	WEEKLY MILEAGE
11	1 mi. easy	3 mi. easy or medium	2 mi. easy	4 mi. easy or medium	2 mi. easy	Rest	5 mi. easy or medium	17
12	2 mi. easy	3 mi. easy or medium	2 mi. easy	4 mi. easy or medium	2 mi. easy	Rest	6 mi. easy or medium	19
13	1 mi. easy	3 mi. easy or medium	2 mi. easy	4 mi. easy or medium	2 mi. easy	Rest	5 mi. easy or medium	17
14	2 mi. easy	3 mi. easy or medium	2 mi. easy	4 mi. easy or medium	2 mi. easy	Rest	6 mi. easy or medium	19
15	Rest	2 mi. easy or medium	1 mi. easy	2 mi. easy or medium	1 mi. easy	Rest	4 mi. easy or medium	10

Cornett also offers programs that move beyond this mileage level for those interested in participating in races ranging from a 5-K to a marathon. (Someone interested in racing might do a 5-K at the end of week 10.) The pattern remains the same; the daily distances continue to increase.

Cornett emphasizes that the route to fitness is not always easy, neither in the beginning nor as you continue. "The first day, people love it," he says. "The second day, they're miserable because their muscles are sore. The third day, they're still miserable because their bodies are still healing. On the fourth day, they begin to feel better. If you can get people to continue in the program at a gentle and easy level, they'll begin to experience all the positive benefits of exercise. Then they're hooked for life."

4

THE 5-K
PADDY SAVAGE'S
FIRST-TIMERS' PROGRAM

Patrick J. Savage coaches not one but three groups of runners. That's in addition to a full-time job as a teacher of business education at Niles West High School in the northwest suburbs of Chicago. Savage, a fiery-haired Irishman who is called Paddy by his friends, not only coaches the boys' track and cross-country teams at Niles West, he also coaches the men's and women's track-and-field teams at nearby Oakton Community College as well as 200 adults who are members of his Niles West/Oakton Runners Club. Add to that his responsibilities as director of the largest high school cross-country meet in the United States, and you have an idea of how dedicated to running Savage is.

In adding that last item to his résumé, Savage remarks that several other cross-country meets in the United States are larger, "but none are sponsored by a high school." Sixty-eight boys' teams and

59 girls' teams participated in the meet in 1996, coming from Wisconsin, Indiana, New York, and Illinois. Originally called the Niles West Invitational, the meet recently was renamed the Patrick J. Savage Invitational, in honor of Paddy himself.

Born in 1944 in a naval hospital in Brooklyn, New York, where his father was stationed during World War II, Savage didn't run during his freshman year at St. Mel's High School in Chicago because he was studying the violin. "My sophomore year, Dean Hayes (now coaching at Middle Tennessee State University and an assistant Olympic coach) talked me into coming out for cross-country." Savage ran 4:37 in the mile and 2:00 in the half-mile, good enough for a scholarship to De Paul University in Chicago.

Savage improved to 9:22 in the two-mile, but a knee injury prevented him from competing in track his senior year of college. His coach, Don Amidei, got him a job teaching and coaching at De Paul Academy. The next year, he moved to St. George High School and finally to Niles West, where he founded his high school invitational in the fall of 1971. He added the Oakton job that same year. "The Oakton runners practice at the high school," Savage explains. "I control the schedules, so I avoid any conflicts."

Supervising two groups of runners should have been enough for any coach, and it was enough for Savage until the mother of one of his runners came to him for help. Her name was Katie Vandergraaf, and she was hoping to improve her times for the 5-K and other road race distances. "Katie kept bugging me," Savage recalls. "She said she had a group of women runners who were looking for a coach. I finally invited them to show up at practice one day."

Savage recalls it as a rainy day in April of 1989. Six other women arrived with Vandergraaf. Scheduled for the day's workout was a warmup jog of a mile, then eight sprints up a hill, another mile jog, six 800-meter repeats on the track, and a mile cooldown. "The rain kept coming down harder," Savage smiles. "Some of my high schoolers started asking when the workout would be over, but none of the women did."

The women practiced weekly with the team for the rest of the school year, then continued with speed workouts through the summer in the evenings. Thus began the Niles West/Oakton Runners Club, which now trains regularly on Monday and Wednesday nights, with races and long runs scheduled on the weekends. The group won the Chicago Area Running Association's club championship seven consecutive years, from 1989 through 1995.

Most people run for fitness, not for competition. Savage, however, feels that the transition from fitness runner to competitive racer can be made painlessly.

Your First 5-K

Savage recommends a 12-week training program that requires running only three days a week. There is a base period of 4 weeks that features walking and jogging for 30 to 45 minutes. "You jog until you become winded, then you walk until you recover," Savage explains. Beginning with the 5th week, Savage's beginners switch their thinking from minutes to miles. The buildup progresses from a run of 1.5 miles to 3 miles over the next 8 weeks, leading to the 5-K race.

Beginning with the ninth week, Savage introduces his beginners to interval training: running repeats of 200 to 800 meters at a medium pace (75 to 80 percent of maximum heart rate) and walking between repeats. This interval workout is preceded by 10 to 15 minutes of walking to warm up, with another 5 to10 minutes of walking afterward to cool down. During the final month before the 5-K race, Savage suggests adding a fourth workout to the week that consists mainly of walking.

The final week before the race, Savage asks his beginners to run their 3-mile run on Tuesday at a slightly faster pace: easy (65 to 75 percent of maximum heart rate). "This is mainly for confidence," Savage explains. "A lot of beginners worry that they won't be able to run 5-K in a race, even though they've been covering that distance in practice."

On race day, Savage tells beginners that their only goal is to finish, running all the way. "I also tell them to be sure to pin their numbers on the fronts of their T-shirts, not the backs," he says. "That way, spectators will recognize them as racers."

After running a 5-K, many runners race no more, or they may enter organized races only sporadically, maybe once a year. "Others enjoy the experience of organized competition, even if they have no desire to race fast," Savage explains. "They like the carnival atmosphere of races and the camaraderie displayed by other middle-of-the-pack runners. Running races and earning more T-shirts become part of their social lives."

Buildup Program

Week	Tues.	Thurs.	Sat.	Sun.
1	30 min. jog or walk	30 min. jog or walk	30 min. jog or walk	Rest
2	35 min. jog or walk	35 min. jog or walk	35 min. jog or walk	Rest
3	40 min. jog or walk	40 min. jog or walk	40 min. jog or walk	Rest
4	45 min. jog or walk	45 min. jog or walk	45 min. jog or walk	Rest
5	1.5 mi. jog	1.5 mi. jog	1.5 mi. jog	Rest
6	1.75 mi. jog	1.75 mi. jog	1.75 mi. jog	Rest
7	2 mi. jog	2 mi. jog	2 mi. jog	Rest
8	2.25 mi. jog	2.25 mi. jog	2.25 mi. jog	Rest
9	2.5 mi. jog	10 x 200 medium	2.5 mi. jog	30 min. walk
10	2.75 mi. jog	8 x 300 medium	2.75 mi. jog	40 min. walk
11	3 mi. jog	6 x 400 medium	3 mi. jog	50 min. walk
12	3 mi. easy	3 x 800 medium	Rest	5-K RACE

Continuing to Race

Savage offers an eight-week training program for beginners who want to continue in racing, perhaps even moving up in distance from the 5-K to another frequently held event, the 8-K (4.96 miles). Not everybody who wants to continue as a runner and participate in occasional road races has time to train daily. The program shown in the table below builds on the one before, with a pattern of two workouts during the middle of the week (Tuesday and Thursday) and two on the weekend (Saturday and Sunday).

Tuesday features a run at jog pace over progressively longer distances. (If you feel strong, you can run the workout slightly faster, at easy pace.) Thursday mimics the interval training in the previous schedule, also progressing in difficulty to 10 × 400 meters in the fourth and eighth weeks. Rather than walking 5 to 10 minutes to

Race-Maintenance Program

WEEK	TUES.	THURS.	SAT.	SUN.
1	3.25 mi. jog or easy	8 x 400 medium	3.25 mi. easy	Cross-train
2	3.5 mi. jog or easy	6 x 600 medium	3.5 mi. easy	Cross-train
3	3.75 mi. jog or easy	4 x 800 medium	3.75 mi. easy	Cross-train
4	4 mi. jog or easy	10 x 400 medium	Rest	5-K RACE
5	4.5 mi. jog or easy	5 x 800 medium	4.5 mi. easy	Cross-train
6	5 mi. jog or easy	12 x 200 medium	5 mi. easy	Cross-train
7	5.5 mi. jog or easy	6 x 800 medium	5.5 mi. easy	Cross-train
8	6 mi. jog or easy	10 x 400 medium	Rest	8-K RACE

warm up and cool down, you will probably want to jog and add some stretching exercises.

Saturday repeats the distance suggested for Tuesday, but at a faster (easy) pace. (If you feel strong, you can pick up the pace in the middle miles to "medium," converting the workout into a tempo run.) On a weekend when you have a 5-K or 8-K race scheduled for Sunday, rest the day before. If you race on Saturday, juggle the schedule accordingly.

Sunday is scheduled as a day of cross-training: an hour of walking, biking, swimming, or even jogging, depending on your mood. If other activities interfere, feel free to juggle workouts from day to day while maintaining the same general training pattern.

This schedule can be maintained indefinitely, depending on your desires and goals. You can remain a fitness runner and still participate in an occasional 5-K or other short road race. If you want to move up to the 10-K or even the marathon, chapters 6 and 9 can help you prepare for your new goals.

5

A FASTER 5-K
ROY BENSON'S
SPEED-IMPROVEMENT PROGRAM

Most beginning runners move quickly up in distance to the point where they complete their first 10-K, a popular racing distance. The next goal for many is the marathon, but Roy Benson, a coach and fitness consultant from Atlanta, believes that runners should look back to consider race distances they've passed en route to running longer and longer. Specifically, he believes that runners need to focus more attention on the 5-K. "If you can improve your speed at shorter distances," he says, "it will help your performances at all distances."

Benson, who was a middle-distance runner in college, served as the track and cross-country coach at the University of Florida before becoming executive director of the Atlanta Track Club, where his duties included directing the Peachtree Road Race. Currently, he coaches more than 100 adult runners by phone and fax and runs a series of running camps from Vermont to California. (For information on the running camps, contact Benson at 5600 Roswell Road, 355N, Atlanta, GA 30342; 404-255-6234.)

Once you have developed the stamina and endurance to not only finish a 10-K but finish it at some selected pace, Benson believes, you are ready to attempt a structured program aimed at improving your baseline speed. He considers the 5-K an ideal distance for speed improvement. "It's short enough so that you can race it frequently without getting hurt," he says, "and it's fast enough so that you need to work on your speed if you expect to achieve success."

Seeking Speed

Coach Benson believes that it takes 8 to 16 weeks for a 10-K runner to convert to a faster 5-K runner. He recommends adding two speed sessions and one stress workout to your weekly training routine.

Interval training. A typical workout would be 12 × 400 meters with 200-meter jogs to rest in between. The 400s should be fast enough to elevate your heart rate to nearly 90 percent of maximum effort, or hard pace. "Heart rates don't elevate immediately," Benson warns. "You don't reach these levels until toward the end of the repeats or toward the end of the workout. So you need to be consistent about when you take your heart rate." The recovery jogs should be slow enough to guarantee that your heart rate drops below 70 percent of maximum, or easy pace. Benson provides the athletes he coaches with pacing charts to aid them in deciding how fast to train. For those without heart rate monitors, he suggests that the training pace be close to race pace, the speed at which you realistically would expect to race your next 5-K.

Speedwork. This second speed session also uses the fast/slow format of interval training, but with shorter distances and speeds at a pace faster than above. A typical workout might be 12 × 200 meters with 200-meter rest jogs between repeats. The 200s should be done fast enough to elevate your heart rate to above 90 percent of maximum effort, or sprint pace. During the recovery jogs, your heart rate drops below 70 percent of maximum. In this workout, Benson's athletes run significantly faster than 5-K pace, closer to 1500-meter (or mile) race pace.

Hill repeats. Hills don't come with standard elevations and distances. Runners usually pick a hill convenient to where they live or train. If you live in a city as flat as Gainesville, Florida, as Marty Liquori did in 1975, when he was ranked first in the world at 5000 meters, you may need to train by running up stadium steps. (That's how Liquori did it.) Benson visualizes the ideal hill as steep enough to force you to breathe hard while powering up but not so steep that you can't maintain some level of speed. It should be long enough so that it takes about a minute to climb. A typical hill workout might include 6 to 10 repeats. "If the hill is 60 seconds or longer, you probably would do about 7 repeats at hard pace," Benson advises. "If you can climb the hill in 45 seconds, you may need to do 10 or more repeats at sprint pace." If the hill takes much longer than 60 seconds to climb, Benson suggests stopping midway up.

Three stress workouts a week are not easy to achieve. For that reason, Benson recommends cutting training mileage. He considers 25 to 30 miles a week suitable for runners who are seeking to improve their 5-K race times, whereas someone more focused on 10-K races might need to run 40 to 45 weekly miles. For those runners who have difficulty fitting three stress workouts into their schedules without experiencing the fatigue that comes with overtraining, Benson cuts their stress workouts to two a week in a 14-day cycle. He alternates the intervals and speedwork from one week to the next, with hill repeats every 7 days.

In guiding experienced 10-K runners who seek to improve their 5-K race speeds, Benson divides his training program into three phases, spaced over a 16-week period.

Phase 1: Base

Don't start at this level if you are a novice runner. This program assumes that you already are fit, have the ability to finish 5-K and 10-K races comfortably, and are looking to do better. Before beginning, you probably should have at least one year's background in which you have included at least some racing in your training program.

During this first phase, Benson programs mile repeats on Tuesday and hill repeats on Thursday. The mile repeats should be run with 400-meter jogs between. During the hill repeats, you simply turn around and jog back down to the bottom of the hill, then start up again. He suggests one or two rest days: a planned day of rest on Monday and an optional day of rest on Friday.

Phase 1

WEEK	MON.	TUES.	WED.	THURS.	FRI.	SAT.	SUN.
1	Rest	1 x 1 mi. crisp	4 mi. easy	5 x hill medium	0–4 mi. easy	2 mi. medium	6 mi. easy
2	Rest	2 x 1 mi. crisp	4 mi. easy	6 x hill medium	0–4 mi. easy	3 mi. medium	7 mi. easy
3	Rest	3 x 1 mi. crisp	4 mi. easy	7 x hill medium	0–4 mi. easy	4 mi. medium	8 mi. easy
4	Rest	4 x 1 mi. crisp	4 mi. easy	8 x hill medium	0–4 mi. easy	5 mi. medium	9 mi. easy

Phase 2: Buildup

In the second phase, mile repeats on Tuesday are replaced by 400 repeats, with 200-meter jogs between repeats. The hill repeats on Thursday are done at a faster pace. A third speed workout is added on Saturday: 200-meter repeats done at a hard pace, jogging 200 meters between. Both to measure fitness and to get mentally ready for the serious racing that begins in phase 3, Benson suggests doing a 10-K race,

Phase 2

WEEK	MON.	TUES.	WED.	THURS.	FRI.	SAT.	SUN.
5	Rest	9 x 400 crisp	4 mi. easy	5 x hill crisp	0–4 mi. easy	9 x 200 hard	5 mi. easy
6	Rest	10 x 400 crisp	4 mi. easy	6 x hill crisp	0–4 mi. easy	10 x 200 hard	6 mi. easy
7	Rest	11 x 400 crisp	4 mi. easy	7 x hill crisp	0–4 mi. easy	**10-K RACE**	7 mi. easy
8	Rest	12 x 400 crisp	4 mi. easy	8 x hill crisp	0–4 mi. easy	12 x 200 hard	8 mi. easy

programmed here in the seventh week. Rest days remain constant. To compensate for the extra speedwork, Sunday runs are slightly shorter.

Phase 3: Racing

In the final phase, competition begins with frequent races on weekends, leading up to a peak 5-K race in the final week. On Tuesday, jog 200 meters between the 400 repeats. On Thursday, run a hill that takes you 45 seconds rather than 60 seconds to climb, permitting a much faster pace. Rest the day before the 5-K races. (If you race on Sunday rather than Saturday, adjust your schedule accordingly.) The final week with its climactic 5-K includes a brief taper.

Phase 3

WEEK	MON.	TUES.	WED.	THURS.	FRI.	SAT.	SUN.
9	Rest	9 x 400 hard	3 mi. easy	6 x hill hard	Rest	**5-K RACE**	4 mi. easy
10	Rest	10 x 400 hard	3 mi. easy	10 x hill hard	3 mi. easy	9 x 200 sprint	6 mi. easy
11	Rest	11 x 400 hard	3 mi. easy	6 x hill hard	Rest	**5-K RACE**	4 mi. easy
12	Rest	12 x 400 hard	3 mi. easy	10 x hill hard	3 mi. easy	10 x 200 sprint	6 mi. easy
13	Rest	9 x 400 hard	3 mi. easy	6 x hill hard	Rest	**5-K RACE**	4 mi. easy
14	Rest	10 x 400 hard	3 mi. easy	6 x hill hard	Rest	**5-K RACE**	4 mi. easy
15	Rest	11 x 400 hard	3 mi. easy	10 x hill hard	3 mi. easy	12 x 200 sprint	6 mi. easy
16	Rest	8 x 200 sprint	3 mi. easy	4 x hill crisp	Rest	**5-K RACE**	Rest

While Benson prescribes target heart rates for individuals whom he coaches, he believes in allowing a wide range for each workout. "As a coach, you need to be intellectually honest," he says. "Some days runners are more fatigued than other days. You need to permit some 'wiggle room.' There are times when an 85 to 95 percent workout should be run at the bottom (85) rather than the top (95). I'd rather have my runners fudge toward the low side, because they're less likely to get injured. If you can train consistently and avoid getting injured, you'll achieve success."

After peaking for this final 5-K—particularly after five races in eight weeks—you probably need to program some rest. Most high school and college coaches tell their runners to take one to two weeks off following an intensive cross-country or track season, and it makes sense for adults, too. Don't worry about losing fitness if you cut back on your training or even do no running at all. The psychological and physical benefits of rest will more than make up for any loss of fitness. One pattern to consider would be to do no running for one week, then easy running the next. During this "down" period, take time to consider your next training and racing goal.

6

THE 10-K
A VERY BASIC
TRAINING PROGRAM

One of the world's most popular road-racing distances is the 10-K, or 10,000 meters, approximately 6.2 miles. The 10,000 meters is also the longest track distance in the Olympic Games. According to the USA Track and Field Road Racing Information Center, 1,522,500 runners participated in 10-K races in the United States in 1996. The event is second in popularity only to the 5-K, which had 2,352,000 finishers the same year.

Soon after completing their first 5-K, many new runners set their sights on double the distance. If that description fits you, here is a basic training program that will allow you to move up to the longer event. This chapter also includes several additional schedules that you can use to help you improve and set a personal record if you're a more experienced runner.

Not much serious training is required—perhaps three or four

workouts a week over a period of several weeks. A weekly average of a dozen miles or so will do the trick. That does not mean you will finish the 10-K well or comfortably, but you will finish.

And you do not necessarily need to run the full distance in practice to prove that you can do it in a race. Most marathoners run no more than 20 miles in workouts before attempting a 26.2-mile race. If you can cover 4 miles in practice several times over a period of weeks and without excessive straining, the spirit of the moment should carry you to the finish line, as long as you start slowly and continue at a comfortable pace.

Tackling the 10-K

Following is a simple eight-week training schedule designed to get you in shape for a 10-K race. Notice that, as is the case for many other training schedules in this book (even those for advanced marathoners), rest is very important. Monday is designed as a rest day. Saturday is what might be called a "cross-training" day elsewhere, mostly light walking. Sunday is the day for the long run—and for a first-time 10-K runner, a run of 1 to 2 miles in the first two weeks does qualify as long.

The middle of the week is when you do some running at shorter distances, just to get used to training on a daily basis. On some of these days, you combine jogging and walking, moving from one mode to the other as your feelings dictate. Is there a difference between a "jog/walk" day and a "walk/jog" day? Yes. On one day you do more jogging than walking, and on the other you do more walking than jogging. You need to be the judge of how much of each you do. Be aware that some days, because of outside pressures at work or at home, you may be more tired than on other days and less in the mood for running. Don't be afraid to adjust your training to accommodate these mood swings. It is what experienced runners call listening to their bodies. On the other hand, you can't compromise your training too much, or you won't be ready to finish that 10-K.

The progression involves an increase in mileage every second week. If you're coming from a low fitness base, having run little before, you

10-K Program for Beginners

WEEK	MON.	TUES.	WED.	THURS.	FRI.	SAT.	SUN.	WEEKLY MILEAGE
1	Rest	1 mi. jog	Light walk	2 mi. jog or walk	1 mi. jog	Light walk	1–2 mi. easy	5–6
2	Rest	1 mi. jog	Light walk	2 mi. jog or walk	1 mi. jog	Light walk	1–2 mi. easy	5–6
3	Rest	2 mi. jog or walk	1 mi. jog	2 mi. easy	1 mi. jog	Light walk	2–3 mi. easy	8–9
4	Rest	2 mi. jog or walk	1 mi. jog	2 mi. easy	1 mi. jog	Light walk	2–3 mi. easy	8–9
5	Rest	2 mi. jog	1 mi. jog	3 mi. jog or walk	2 mi. jog	Light walk or jog	3–4 mi. easy	11–12
6	Rest	2 mi. jog	1 mi. jog	3 mi. jog or walk	2 mi. jog	Light walk or jog	3–4 mi. easy	11–12
7	Rest	3 mi. jog or walk	2 mi. jog	3 mi. easy	2 mi. jog	Light walk or jog	4 mi. easy	14
8	Rest	3 mi. jog or walk	2 mi. jog	3 mi. easy	Light walk or jog	Rest	**10-K RACE**	14

may want to take more than the eight weeks prescribed to prepare for your first 10-K. Simply repeat any one of the weeks at any point in the schedule. On days when the training plan suggests light walking or jogging, cover whatever distance seems appropriate to the way you feel. A mile or two should be sufficient. Unless you have some specific hometown 10-K that you hope to run, you usually can find any number of 10-K races for your first attempt at this distance. Specific goals, though, can help motivate you. Most people will want to focus on a particular 10-K as the end of their training rainbow.

This same training program can be used by beginners to prepare for races of distances shorter than 10-K. If that local race you want to run is a 5-K or 8-K, for example, you can still use this schedule.

Notice that in the final week, you have two easy days leading to your first 10-K race. It is always important to go to the starting line of any major race well-rested. Following your first 10-K, take a day or two off. You will have earned your rest. Then you can set your sights on your next running goal.

Training to Improve Your 10-K Times

To enjoy continued success in 10-K races and to improve your times, you need to do more training than that suggested in the training program for beginners. Don't just run more miles; run them faster. If you are an experienced runner who is looking to improve your 10-K times, you may have skipped the preceding paragraphs. The following charts and schedules are designed for you.

The late Fred Wilt, who ran the 10,000 meters in the 1948 and 1952 Olympic Games and later coached the women's cross-country and track-and-field teams at Purdue University in Indiana, felt that the route to 10-K success required runners to do at least some speedwork. He once wrote, "For top results in the 10,000 meters, training should be about the same for both road and track. But road runners often do not put in sufficient high-speed, anaerobic training. Specifically, they do not do enough repetitions at a speed equal to, or slightly faster than, the best average time they expect to run in competition." Wilt believed that this type of running should be done once or twice a week. He also believed in daily sprints: three to six 50- to 100-meter dashes done at the end of the warmup, before the major part of the workout.

"Most good road runners put in sufficient mileage to race 10,000 meters," Wilt said. "The only problem is that they should carefully monitor the quality (speed) of their running if they want to produce their best results." He felt that correct 10-K training should include about 80 percent aerobic (easy) running and 20 percent anaerobic (hard) running. An infinite number of training variations are possible using this 80/20 ratio.

No ideal method of training exists for either the 10-K or other distances. People's abilities to adapt to hard work differ. Nevertheless, basic training techniques are the same for everybody, men and women, teenagers and masters. Whether you train on the road, on a track, or on trails probably doesn't matter. The most important factors for success in improving your 10-K times are your desire and your willingness to follow a training program in which you mix intensity and volume. Proper rest is also important, particularly before you race.

The following table offers guidelines for 10-K runners who want to design their own training programs. You can place yourself in the appropriate category depending on your best times for the mile or 10-K. Column 3 tells you your approximate 10-K race pace per mile based on your best 10-K time. Columns 4 and 5 suggest how many miles to train a week and the length of your longest workout. Column 6 advises how many speed sessions to run weekly. Columns 7 and 8 tell you how fast to run 400 meters in workouts, running a small number at sprint pace or a larger number at hard pace. Remember that this chart is intended only as a guide. Your actual training times may vary depending on your basic speed and level of fitness.

10-K Training Guidelines

Category	Best Time: 10-K	Best Time: Mile	Pace per Mile: 10-K	Weekly Mileage	Longest Workout	Weekly Speed Sessions	Sprint Speed: 400 Meters	Hard Speed: 400 Meters
Novice	49:30	6:38	8:00	20	6–9 mi.	1	1:40	2:00
Inter-mediate I	43:30	5:48	7:00	30	8–10 mi.	1–2	1:27	1:40
Inter-mediate II	37:00	5:04	6:00	45	10–14 mi.	2	1:16	1:30
Expert	31:00	4:16	5:00	80	14–20 mi.	3	1:04	1:15

Workout Patterns

Category	Mon.	Tues.	Wed.	Thurs.	Fri.	Sat.	Sun.
Novice	Rest	1 mi. wup (jog); 8 x 400 (hard), walking between 400s; 1 mi. cdn (jog)	4 mi. easy	1 mi. wup (jog); 3 x 400 (sprint), walking between 400s; 1 mi. cdn (jog)	4 mi. easy	2 mi. jog	4 mi. easy
Inter-mediate I	2 mi. jog	1 mi. wup (jog); 10 x 400 (hard), walking between 400s; 1 mi. cdn (jog)	4 mi. easy	30 min. fartlek	6 mi. easy	2 mi. easy	10 mi. easy
Inter-mediate II	4 mi. jog	1 mi. wup (jog); 12 x 400 (hard), jogging between 400s; 1 mi. cdn (jog)	6 mi. easy	1 mi. wup (jog); 4 x 400 (sprint), walking between 400s; 1 mi. cdn (jog)	9 mi. easy	4 mi. easy	14 mi. easy
Expert	10 mi. easy	3 mi. wup (jog); 16 x 400 (hard), jogging between 400s; 2 mi. cdn (jog)	12 mi. easy	3 mi. wup (jog); 4–5 x 400 (sprint), walking between 400s; 2 mi. cdn (jog)	9 mi. easy	60 min. fartlek	20 mi. easy

Progression

The schedules on the opposite page offer some training patterns for different experience levels. As you become more fit over time, you probably won't want to repeat the same workouts week after week. So consider the schedules as something to shoot for at the peak of your program, what you want to be doing right before your most important 10-K race. You may want to begin your training at one or two levels below your peak level and work toward that goal. For example, intermediate runners can begin with the novice schedule and work gradually toward their training goals. But be flexible with your training, and don't be afraid to take extra rest days or rest weeks.

Following is an example of how a runner at the Intermediate II level might progress with his training over a period of six weeks. He would begin in week 1 with the training pattern used by Intermediate I runners. Each week, he would run a little bit farther until he reached his peak week, which has 14 miles as its longest run (the pattern for Intermediate II). It might be necessary to modify this schedule to accommodate training for races at 10-K or other distances.

Sample Progression

WEEK	MON.	TUES.	WED.	THURS.	FRI.	SAT.	SUN.
1	2 mi. jog	10 x 400 hard	4 mi. easy	30 min. fartlek	6 mi. easy	2 mi. easy	10 mi. easy
2	2 mi. jog	10 x 400 hard	5 mi. easy	3 x 400 sprint	7 mi. easy	2 mi. easy	11 mi. easy
3	3 mi. jog	11 x 400 hard	5 mi. easy	35 min. fartlek	7 mi. easy	3 mi. easy	12 mi. easy
4	3 mi. jog	11 x 400 hard	5 mi. easy	3 x 400 sprint	8 mi. easy	3 mi. easy	13 mi. easy
5	4 mi. jog	12 x 400 hard	6 mi. easy	40 min. fartlek	8 mi. easy	4 mi. easy	14 mi. easy
6	4 mi. jog	12 x 400 hard	6 mi. easy	4 x 400 sprint	9 mi. easy	4 mi. easy	**10-K RACE**

7

THE HALF-MARATHON
MOVING UP (OR DOWN)
TO 13.1 MILES

Two favorite racing distances among runners are the 10-K and the marathon. Thus, individuals who decide to train for a half-marathon often approach that race of 13.1 miles (21.1 kilometers) from one end or the other. If they have been running mostly 10-K races, they have to race farther and slower. Coming from the marathon, they have to race shorter and faster.

Gearing Up

Let's say you're running 25 to 30 miles a week and have just finished several months of mostly 10-K races. Now you have your eyes set on a half-marathon in five weeks, either for its own sake or as a stepping stone to an eventual marathon. A well-trained runner who has raced in

5-K and/or 10-K races should be able to move up in distance with five weeks of specialized training, but what should this training be?

Using the table below, you can increase your training mileage to prepare for this longer distance. For the tempo run scheduled for Tuesday, do the first and last mile easy and the middle miles between medium and crisp. The 10-K race scheduled at the end of the third week is to aid you in predicting your half-marathon time.

One important word of advice about the buildup in miles leading to the half-marathon: If you want to go *farther*, you can do so more easily by running *slower*.

Gearing Up for the Half-Marathon

WEEK	MON.	TUES.	WED.	THURS.	FRI.	SAT.	SUN.
1	Rest	4 mi. easy	6 mi. easy	4 mi. easy	6 mi. medium	4 mi. easy	7 mi. easy
2	Rest	4 mi. tempo	6 mi. easy	4 mi. easy	7 mi. medium	4 mi. easy	8 mi. easy
3	Rest	4 mi. tempo	6 mi. easy	5 mi. easy	7 mi. medium	Rest	10-K RACE
4	Rest	4 mi. easy	6 mi. easy	6 mi. easy	8 mi. medium	4 mi. easy	10 mi. easy
5	Rest	5 mi. tempo	6 mi. easy	5 mi. easy	3 mi. jog	Rest	HALF-MARATHON

Gearing Down

You're running 50 to 60 miles a week and have recently completed a marathon. Now, after having taken several weeks off to recuperate and to keep motivated, you would like to try a race at the less stressful half-marathon distance. How should you train?

Here is how, during a five-week period, you might increase the quality of your training to prepare for the shorter (thus faster) half-marathon distance. One important, if obvious, piece of advice: If you want to go *faster*, you can do so more easily by *cutting your mileage*.

You also need to do some speedwork to get used to racing at a faster pace. The following schedule suggests 1-mile repeats on Tuesday and interval training featuring 400 repeats on Thursday. Walk and/or jog for 3 to 5 minutes between repeats. Begin and end each session with a warmup/cooldown jog of 800 to 1600 meters. Also, do some stretching and stride a few 100-meter straightaways to prepare yourself to run fast.

Gearing Down to the Half-Marathon

WEEK	MON.	TUES.	WED.	THURS.	FRI.	SAT.	SUN.
1	Rest	3 x 1 mi. crisp	6 mi. easy	6 x 400 hard	5 mi. easy	6 mi. medium	14 mi. easy
2	Rest	4 x 1 mi. crisp	6 mi. easy	7 x 400 hard	5 mi. easy	8 mi. medium	12 mi. easy
3	Rest	3 x 1 mi. crisp	6 mi. easy	8 x 400 hard	5 mi. easy	Rest	**10-K RACE**
4	Rest	4 x 1 mi. crisp	6 mi. easy	9 x 400 hard	5 mi. easy	4 mi. easy	10 mi. easy
5	Rest	3 x 1 mi. crisp	6 mi. easy	10 x 400 hard	3 mi. jog	Rest	**HALF- MARATHON**

How Fast Can You Run a Half?

Most runners can tell you to a tenth of a second their fastest times for the 5-K, 10-K, or marathon, road racing's most popular distances. They are more vague when citing half-marathon bests, because often they don't give that intermediate distance the attention it deserves. Or they don't run it while in peak condition. Or maybe they've never run it at all.

The table on page 47 allows you to predict how fast you should be able to run 13.1 miles, based on recent 10-K and/or marathon times. The final column reveals how fast you will need to run per mile to hit that time. A cautionary note: Depending upon the amount of speed or endurance you possess, your 10-K and marathon times may not be "equal" as judged by the table. If so, you will need to interpolate.

Prediction Table

10-K Time	Marathon Time	Predicted Half-Marathon Time	Mile Pace for Half-Marathon
27:30	2:08	1:01:15	4:40
30:00	2:20	1:07:00	5:05
32:30	2:32	1:12:30	5:30
35:00	2:44	1:18:15	6:00
37:30	2:56	1:23:45	6:25
40:00	3:09	1:30:00	6:50
42:30	3:21	1:34:45	7:15
45:00	3:33	1:41:00	7:40
50:00	3:58	1:52:30	8:35
55:00	4:23	2:04:30	9:30
60:00	4:48	2:16:00	10:20
70:00	6:00	2:40:00	12:20

SOURCE: *RunningTrax: Computerized Running Training Programs*, by J. Gerry Purdy

8

THE 25-K
GREG MEYER'S
OLD KENT RIVER
BANK PROGRAM

Greg Meyer is a Grand Rapids boy. He was born in that city in south-central Michigan, and he won three state championships (cross-country twice, the mile once) while attending West Catholic High School there. At the University of Michigan, he made All-American four times, graduating in 1977. Meyer's track specialty was the 3000-meter steeplechase, an event that he ran in the 1976 and 1980 Olympic Trials.

He achieved greater success after moving from the track to the road. After running against Bill Rodgers in the first Old Kent River Bank Run, held in Grand Rapids in 1978, Meyer accepted an invitation to move to Boston and train with the Greater Boston Track Club, then coached by Bill Squires. Meyer worked part-time in Rodgers's running store, located at Cleveland Circle, near the 22-mile mark on the Boston Marathon course. In 1983, he won that race in 2:09:00, which is still among the fastest marathon times run by an American. He also won major marathons in Rio de Janeiro and Chicago.

Yet Greg Meyer never forgot his Grand Rapids roots, returning each May to participate in the Old Kent River Bank Run, a 25-K (15.6-mile) race with annual fields of more than 3,000 runners. Meyer has won the River Bank Run on seven occasions. His winning time of 1:14:29 in 1979 was an American record.

A Challenging Course

The Old Kent River Bank Run begins and ends in downtown Grand Rapids. The scenic, tree-shaded course follows the left bank of the Grand River and returns on the right bank, after crossing the Wilson Avenue Bridge about halfway through the course. "It's a challenging course that has three separate segments," Meyer says. "The first segment is the run to the bridge. It's flat and fast. You get a chance to find a smooth rhythm.

"The real racing starts at the bridge," he continues. "After a couple of miles, you move up from the river for a series of hills that last through 12 miles. That's the second segment. The final segment is the 3-mile sprint to the finish. The hills come at you just when you begin to feel fatigued, so it's not only a challenge to go the distance for beginners, it's also a challenge for experienced runners to run it well. Also, the 25-K is a unique distance. It's still a long way from the 26 miles 385 yards of a marathon, meaning that you don't get beaten up too badly, but you need to do some long-distance training beyond what you do for 5-K and 10-K races."

To help runners prepare for the race, Meyer developed a training program in conjunction with the sponsoring Old Kent Bank. "It's a very basic program, designed for beginners," he explains. "It starts with mostly walking but peaks 16 weeks later at about 30 miles a week. If you follow the plan, it will get you to the finish line."

Meyer doesn't recommend a specific training pace but says only to run at a pace that feels comfortable. "If you can't converse with your training partner, you're going too fast," he says. This would suggest a pace equal to easy, or 65 to 75 percent of maximum heart rate.

Twenty-five kilometers is close enough in distance to the more frequently contested half-marathon (21.1 kilometers) that runners training for that distance also can use the 25-K schedule, stopping their mileage buildup after week 12. "The key to the program is the long run scheduled for Saturday. Be consistent with your training, and you'll have no trouble running Old Kent or other races at similar distances," Meyer states.

The Program

For the benefit of runners of different abilities, Meyer has broken his 25-K training program into four phases. The first four-week phase is only for beginning runners—people who have not run before.

Phase 1: Base Training

WEEK	MON.	TUES.	WED.	THURS.	FRI.	SAT.	SUN.	WEEKLY TOTALS
1	20 min. walk	20 min. walk	10 min. walk 3 min. jog 4 min. walk 3 min. jog 5 min. walk	25 min. walk or rest	10 min. walk 3 min. jog 5 min. walk 5 min. jog 7 min. walk	10 min. walk 10 min. jog 10 min. walk	25 min. walk or rest	24 min. jogging
2	10 min. walk 5 min. jog 5 min. walk	10 min. walk 10 min. jog 10 min. walk	10 min. walk 5 min. jog 5 min. walk	25 min. walk or rest	10 min. walk 5 min. jog 5 min. walk	10 min. walk 15 min. jog 10 min. walk	30 min. walk or rest	40 min. jogging
3	10 min. walk 10 min. jog 10 min. walk	10 min. walk 15 min. jog 10 min. walk	35 min. walk or rest	10 min. walk 15 min. jog 10 min. walk	10 min. walk 10 min. jog 10 min. walk	5 min. walk 20 min. jog 5 min. walk	35 min. walk or rest	70 min. jogging
4	1 mi. run	1.5 mi. run	2 mi. run	30 min. walk or rest	1 mi. run	3 mi. run	30 min. walk or rest	8.5 mi. running

Meyer recommends that runners be examined by a qualified physician before beginning this schedule. "It is your responsibility to determine that you are fit enough to undertake this program and to monitor its effects on your health," he warns. Experienced runners will probably want to skip this phase and jump forward to phase 2, which begins in the program's fifth week.

Meyer suggests that the walking should be "brisk." Jogging should be done at a slow pace, or what is listed as "jog" in our Universal Pace Chart (see page 9).

Phase 2: Mileage Buildup

WEEK	MON.	TUES.	WED.	THURS.	FRI.	SAT.	SUN.	WEEKLY MILEAGE
5	1.5 mi. run	2 mi. run	3 mi. run	1 mi. jog or rest	2 mi. run	4 mi. run	1 mi. jog or rest	12.5–14.5
6	2 mi. run	1 mi. run	4 mi. run	1 mi. jog or rest	2 mi. run	5 mi. run	1.5 mi. jog or rest	14–16.5
7	3 mi. run	1.5 mi. run	5 mi. run	1.5 mi. jog or rest	2 mi. run	6 mi. run	2 mi. jog or rest	17.5–21
8	4 mi. run	2 mi. run	5 mi. run	2 mi. jog or rest	2 mi. run	7 mi. run	2 mi. jog or rest	20–24
9	3 mi. run	2 mi. run	5 mi. run	2 mi. jog or rest	3 mi. run	8 mi. run	2 mi. jog or rest	21–25
10	4 mi. run	2 mi. run	5 mi. run	2 mi. jog or rest	2 mi. run	9 mi. run	2 mi. jog or rest	22–26
11	2 mi. run	6 mi. run	3 mi. run	2 mi. jog or rest	2 mi. run	10 mi. run	2 mi. jog or rest	23–27
12	3 mi. run	2 mi. run	6 mi. run	2 mi. jog or rest	3 mi. run	11 mi. run	2 mi. jog or rest	25–29

The end of the four-week base is a good point for evaluating how well you are progressing with your training. "If you cannot physically complete the first four weeks," Meyer says, "you may need to re-evaluate whether you should compete in a 25-K race so soon after beginning training."

Phase 2, shown in the table on page 51, concentrates on mileage buildup. And there's no more walking; all of the workouts during this phase involve running. On Thursday and Sunday, Meyer offers the option of taking the day off or doing what he refers to as an easy run, what we would describe as jog pace.

Here is where runners with previous base endurance may want to enter the program. Even though you might average between 15 and 25 miles a week, you may want to step backward in distance and begin with the week 5 level of 12.5 miles a week to ensure that you are well-rested when you begin the training program.

This phase of the program is not designed for more experienced runners, those who train more than 25 miles weekly and compete regularly in marathons. "The focus is on people doing their first race at a 25-K distance," Meyer says. He suggests, however, that experienced runners can follow this phase of the program by converting the Monday workout into a tempo run with the middle miles at a fast pace, between medium and crisp. Thursday could be for speedwork: hill repeats, or intervals on the track.

If you are planning on racing a half-marathon rather than a 25-K, you may find that you want to plan your schedule so that you race at the end of week 12. But you can still train for the same number of weeks that you might for a 25-K. To do this, simply repeat some of the weeks. Meyer recommends that you repeat weeks 5, 7, 9, and 11 and use the race taper in phase 4 (but with slightly reduced mileage) for your final week.

Phase 3 is where the most serious training occurs. In many respects, the first 12 weeks have been a prelude to this point. The mileage reaches a peak in weeks 15, 16, and 17, and your longest run, 14 miles (done twice), is just short of the race distance.

Phase 3: Race Peaking

Week	Mon.	Tues.	Wed.	Thurs.	Fri.	Sat.	Sun.	Weekly Mileage
13	3 mi. run	6 mi. run	4 mi. run	2 mi. jog or rest	2 mi. run	12 mi. run	2 mi. jog or rest	27–31
14	4 mi. run	2 mi. run	6 mi. run	2 mi. jog or rest	2 mi. run	13 mi. run	2 mi. jog or rest	27–31
15	5 mi. run	3 mi. run	6 mi. run	2 mi. jog or rest	2 mi. run	14 mi. run	2 mi. jog or rest	30–34
16	5 mi. run	2 mi. run	7 mi. run	2 mi. jog or rest	3 mi. run	13 mi. run	2 mi. jog or rest	30–34
17	4 mi. run	3 mi. run	6 mi. run	2 mi. jog or rest	2 mi. run	14 mi. run	2 mi. jog or rest	29–33
18	4 mi. run	3 mi. run	6 mi. run	2 mi. jog or rest	3 mi. run	10 mi. run	2 mi. jog or rest	26–30

All of the serious training has been completed in the three phases above. The final week allows you to taper your training so that you will enter the race well-rested and ready to run.

Phase 4: Race Week

Week	Mon.	Tues.	Wed.	Thurs.	Fri.	Sat.	Sun.	Weekly Mileage
RACE	3 mi. run	5 mi. run	3 mi. run	2 mi. jog or rest	2 mi. run	25-K RACE	Rest	28.5–30.5

Now that you've finished a 25-K, would you like to run farther? You may want to back off your training for two to four weeks to recover. Then, check the marathon training schedules on pages 54 and 66.

9

THE MARATHON
BRIAN PIPER'S CHICAGO MARATHON PROGRAM

In 1989, Brian Piper, a computer systems analyst and 2:58 marathoner from Chicago, organized a four-month training class to prepare local runners to run 26 miles 385 yards. "I had made every mistake imaginable in learning how to run the marathon, and I thought others might benefit by not having to repeat my errors," he says.

Piper patterned his program on one originally developed by the St. Louis Track Club for the marathon in that city. Thirty-five runners enrolled in his first class, organized under the auspices of the Chicago Area Running Association (CARA). By 1997, the class had grown to nearly 750 runners training in eight different locations in and around the city to prepare for The LaSalle Banks Chicago Marathon in October.

By then, I had become involved in the program as a training consultant along with Bill Fitzgerald, another local marathoner, who helped Piper with the logistics. The class used my *Marathon: The Ultimate Training and Racing Guide* as its textbook. But the program achieved its success because of the many group leaders and volunteers. Members of the class who were doing their long runs at 9:00, or 10:00, or whatever mile pace had others to run with, and experienced group leaders kept them moving at the right speeds and ensured that they stopped often enough to take liquids. It was a very hands-on experience, and it made training for the marathon fun. I particularly enjoyed working with the beginners, who normally made up about 50 percent of the class. A large number were young women, contradicting a belief among the media that marathoners are mostly aging baby boomers. Their excitement was contagious.

Each year's class lasted 18 weeks and consisted of instructional clinics in midweek and long runs on weekends. In addition to my book, enrollees received a booklet that contained our 18-week training schedule. This schedule first appeared in a July 1994 article that I had written for *Runner's World* magazine. It was basically Piper's schedule. Several years after the article appeared, I posted the schedule on my Web site (http://www.halhigdon.com). As soon as I did, traffic to my Web site doubled almost overnight. A lot of runners were looking for a good marathon training schedule.

It is with some pride that I offer you Brian Piper's Chicago Marathon Program. While I was working on this chapter, I called Piper to ask him who deserves credit for the schedules. Usually each spring, Piper, Fitzgerald, and I meet to plan the class, often fine-tuning the schedules to that year's needs. I wasn't sure who should claim authorship. Piper explained that while the inspiration came from St. Louis, he had drafted the original schedule for Chicago with its mileage buildup, but I had provided the day-by-day mileage breakdown for my article in *Runner's World*. Fitzgerald was also working with us to develop the program, but perhaps most of the credit should go to the several thousand runners who trained for Chicago and other marathons in the CARA program. Certainly, we have learned as much from them as they have learned from us.

The program is offered for four levels of runners. The novice schedule is designed for beginners who are seeking to finish their first marathon. Two intermediate schedules (I and II) are for experienced marathoners who are trying to improve their times. The expert schedule is for those marathoners who may have plateaued and want to fine-tune their training, perhaps to qualify for Boston or to set a new personal record.

Focusing on Your Goal

We offer an important message for those entering our program: If you care enough to train for18 weeks to run a marathon, you should focus your training toward that marathon goal. You should set aside or postpone other activities and avoid other stresses. This includes excessive speedwork or racing. Every year at the first class session, people raise their hands during the question-and-answer period and ask for our permission to race in events leading up to the marathon. (You won't see any races listed in the schedules that follow.) CARA has a race circuit with weekly races in which runners score points toward a year-end championship. And inevitably, someone also will ask if it's okay to compete in a popular triathlon held in Chicago in midsummer.

We don't say yes; we don't say no. Our class consists of consenting adults, and we can't deny them TV-watching privileges for the week after catching them in a triathlon. But we do warn that too much racing can compromise their training, because racing interferes with the long runs that are planned for each weekend and are the core of the program. In fact, if you did little more than one long workout each weekend, you could probably complete a marathon, although I don't advise that strategy.

Some racing actually is important for runners who are training for a marathon. Running an occasional race allows you to gauge fitness. Knowing how fast you can run a 10-K helps when it comes time to select a marathon pace. (One formula suggests multiplying your 10-K time in minutes by 4.66 to predict your marathon time.) During our 18-week program, we suggest that participants run no more than three races, spacing them a month or so apart. If and when they do race, we also recommend that they get ample rest before and after. This means cutting back slightly on mileage during race weeks. Our program features regular step-backs in mileage every three weeks, so those weeks are best for racing. If the schedule doesn't match their personal race calendar, we ask them to be flexible in shifting workouts from week to week while maintaining the integrity of the mileage buildup.

The longest training run in our program is 20 miles, run once by beginners and slightly more often by those with more experience. Seven-time Boston Marathon champion Clarence DeMar once told another Boston legend, Johnny Kelley, "You have to run 20-milers to get ready for the marathon, but you don't want to run too many of them." That advice still makes sense a half-century later.

One question that is frequently asked by beginners—and some experienced runners—is, "How can you expect to run 26 miles 385 yards in a race if you never run that far in practice?" Many major marathons have training programs that are just as successful as ours in Chicago. In Portland Bob Williams (working with Warren and Patti Fink) takes runners up to 22 miles for their longest run. Jeff Galloway offers marathon training programs in many cities with 26 miles (walking breaks included) as his ultimate practice goal. In Minnesota Bill Wenmark sometimes takes experienced runners as far as 31 miles while preparing them for the Twin Cities Marathon or Grandma's Marathon. In Texas Robert Vaughan thinks in minutes rather than miles, with 4 hours the max for those who train under his direction for the Dallas White Rock Marathon.

You can't separate any one individual workout from the totality of the program, however, and each of these respected coaches has found success doing things his way. In Chicago, we feel that if you can run 20 miles in practice, the inspiration of running in a field of 15,000 like-minded runners will carry you that extra 6 miles, 385 yards on race day, particularly if you taper the last two to three weeks and enter the race well-rested.

It has worked for us, and hopefully the following marathon training programs will work for you.

Novice Schedule

We like beginners who enter our program to already be running three to four days a week, totaling 15 to 20 miles a week. Hopefully, they will have run several previous races at 5-K or 10-K distances. If they are not at that level, they may want to postpone their marathon plans. Every year we have anxious runners who enter our program and then realize as the miles continue to build relentlessly that they may have overestimated their base level of conditioning. We tell them to continue to train at a slightly reduced level and see us the following year. If you spend *at least* a year getting in shape and developing a base level of fitness before attempting your first marathon, it will make the experience much more enjoyable.

First-time marathoners should both train and race conservatively. The following 18-week training schedule tells you simply how many miles to run each day. The week's work divides into four phases.

Base (Tuesday, Wednesday, Thursday). Midweek runs should be run at easy pace. If you feel good, run slightly faster (medium) on Wednesday, but don't overdo it.

Rest (Monday, Friday). Friday's rest day is to get ready for the weekend long run; Monday's rest day is for recovery. Rest is a *very* important part of the training program.

Distance (Saturday). A long run is scheduled for Saturday but can be done any day. Run at the pace at which you hope to run the marathon—although we always tell first-timers to choose a conservative goal time. Don't hesitate to walk. As a first-timer, your goal should be to finish, not to run fast.

Aerobics (Sunday). A day of active rest. Spend an hour doing some easy cross-training like walking, cycling, or swimming, but usually no running.

Key to the novice marathon training program is the mileage buildup, particularly the long runs. Their lengths increase at a rate of 1 mile per week, from 6 miles in week 1 to 20 miles in week 16. (Taper two weeks before the marathon.) Every third week features a step-back for recovery, for psychological as well as physical reasons. It's a lot easier to do that

	Novice						
WEEK	**MON.**	**TUES.**	**WED.**	**THURS.**	**FRI.**	**SAT.**	**SUN.**
1	Rest	3 mi.	3 mi.	3 mi.	Rest	6 mi.	Aerobics
2	Rest	3 mi.	3 mi.	3 mi.	Rest	7 mi.	Aerobics
3	Rest	3 mi.	4 mi.	3 mi.	Rest	5 mi.	Aerobics
4	Rest	3 mi.	4 mi.	3 mi.	Rest	9 mi.	Aerobics
5	Rest	3 mi.	5 mi.	3 mi.	Rest	10 mi.	Aerobics
6	Rest	3 mi.	5 mi.	3 mi.	Rest	7 mi.	Aerobics
7	Rest	3 mi.	6 mi.	3 mi.	Rest	12 mi.	Aerobics
8	Rest	3 mi.	6 mi.	4 mi.	Rest	13 mi.	Aerobics
9	Rest	3 mi.	7 mi.	4 mi.	Rest	10 mi.	Aerobics
10	Rest	3 mi.	7 mi.	4 mi.	Rest	15 mi.	Aerobics
11	Rest	4 mi.	8 mi.	4 mi.	Rest	16 mi.	Aerobics
12	Rest	4 mi.	8 mi.	5 mi.	Rest	12 mi.	Aerobics
13	Rest	4 mi.	9 mi.	5 mi.	Rest	18 mi.	Aerobics
14	Rest	5 mi.	9 mi.	5 mi.	Rest	19 mi.	Aerobics
15	Rest	5 mi.	10 mi.	5 mi.	Rest	14 mi.	Aerobics
16	Rest	5 mi.	8 mi.	5 mi.	Rest	20 mi.	Aerobics
17	Rest	4 mi.	6 mi.	4 mi.	Rest	8 mi.	Aerobics
18	Rest	3 mi.	4 mi.	Rest	Rest	Rest	**MARATHON**

16-mile run in the 11th week if you know that you need to run only 12 miles the following weekend.

The total weekly mileage progresses in a similar fashion. The program for first-timers is designed for you to run approximately as many total miles midweek as on your long run on the weekend. If you follow the program, doing neither too much nor too little, success in your first marathon is guaranteed.

Intermediate Schedules

Experienced marathoners may want to increase their training with a goal of improving their finishing times. In our Chicago class we offer two intermediate schedules with minor variations between them, recognizing the fact that the largest number of marathoners could be classified as intermediates. Whether a runner picks one or the other is largely a matter of choice, based on his level of experience. The following 18-week training schedules expand upon that offered to beginners. The week's work divides into six phases.

Aerobics (Monday). A day of active rest. Spend 30 to 60 minutes doing some easy cross-training like walking, cycling, or swimming, but usually no running. This is part of your recovery from the weekend long run. Don't overdo it.

Base (Tuesday, Thursday). These short runs should be run at easy pace.

Tempo (Wednesday). Begin and end the tempo run at easy pace with 15 to 30 minutes running at medium to crisp pace in the middle. At the peak of the workout, you should be running at marathon pace or slightly faster.

Rest (Friday). Relax to get ready for the harder training planned for the weekend. Rest remains a very important part of the training program.

Pace (Saturday). Begin and finish easy, but otherwise run the pace at which you plan to race the marathon, or slightly slower. In other words, don't run quite as fast as during Wednesday's tempo run. Save some energy for Sunday's long run.

Distance (Sunday). A long run for intermediate runners is scheduled for Sunday but can be done any day. Run 1 to 2 minutes slower than the pace at which you plan to run the marathon. Just cover the distance; don't worry about time. This should not be a punishing workout.

Key to the intermediate programs, along with the mileage buildup, is the addition of faster runs twice during the week. The long runs also

Intermediate I							
WEEK	**MON.**	**TUES.**	**WED.**	**THURS.**	**FRI.**	**SAT.**	**SUN.**
1	Aerobics	3 mi.	5 mi.	3 mi.	Rest	5 mi.	8 mi.
2	Aerobics	3 mi.	5 mi.	3 mi.	Rest	5 mi.	9 mi.
3	Aerobics	3 mi.	5 mi.	3 mi.	Rest	5 mi.	6 mi.
4	Aerobics	3 mi.	6 mi.	3 mi.	Rest	6 mi.	11 mi.
5	Aerobics	3 mi.	6 mi.	3 mi.	Rest	6 mi.	12 mi.
6	Aerobics	3 mi.	5 mi.	3 mi.	Rest	6 mi.	9 mi.
7	Aerobics	3 mi.	7 mi.	3 mi.	Rest	7 mi.	14 mi.
8	Aerobics	4 mi.	7 mi.	4 mi.	Rest	7 mi.	15 mi.
9	Aerobics	4 mi.	5 mi.	4 mi.	Rest	7 mi.	11 mi.
10	Aerobics	4 mi.	8 mi.	4 mi.	Rest	8 mi.	17 mi.
11	Aerobics	4 mi.	8 mi.	4 mi.	Rest	8 mi.	18 mi.
12	Aerobics	5 mi.	5 mi.	5 mi.	Rest	8 mi.	13 mi.
13	Aerobics	5 mi.	8 mi.	5 mi.	Rest	5 mi.	20 mi.
14	Aerobics	5 mi.	5 mi.	5 mi.	Rest	8 mi.	12 mi.
15	Aerobics	5 mi.	8 mi.	5 mi.	Rest	5 mi.	20 mi.
16	Aerobics	5 mi.	6 mi.	5 mi.	Rest	4 mi.	12 mi.
17	Aerobics	4 mi.	5 mi.	4 mi.	Rest	3 mi.	8 mi.
18	Aerobics	3 mi.	4 mi.	Rest	Rest	1–3 mi.	**MARATHON**

Intermediate II

WEEK	MON.	TUES.	WED.	THURS.	FRI.	SAT.	SUN.
1	Aerobics	3 mi.	5 mi.	3 mi.	Rest	5 mi.	10 mi.
2	Aerobics	3 mi.	5 mi.	3 mi.	Rest	5 mi.	11 mi.
3	Aerobics	3 mi.	6 mi.	3 mi.	Rest	6 mi.	8 mi.
4	Aerobics	3 mi.	6 mi.	3 mi.	Rest	6 mi.	13 mi.
5	Aerobics	3 mi.	7 mi.	3 mi.	Rest	7 mi.	14 mi.
6	Aerobics	3 mi.	7 mi.	3 mi.	Rest	7 mi.	10 mi.
7	Aerobics	3 mi.	8 mi.	3 mi.	Rest	8 mi.	16 mi.
8	Aerobics	4 mi.	8 mi.	4 mi.	Rest	8 mi.	17 mi.
9	Aerobics	4 mi.	9 mi.	4 mi.	Rest	9 mi.	12 mi.
10	Aerobics	4 mi.	9 mi.	4 mi.	Rest	9 mi.	19 mi.
11	Aerobics	4 mi.	10 mi.	4 mi.	Rest	10 mi.	20 mi.
12	Aerobics	5 mi.	6 mi.	5 mi.	Rest	6 mi.	12 mi.
13	Aerobics	5 mi.	10 mi.	5 mi.	Rest	10 mi.	20 mi.
14	Aerobics	5 mi.	6 mi.	5 mi.	Rest	6 mi.	12 mi.
15	Aerobics	5 mi.	10 mi.	5 mi.	Rest	10 mi.	20 mi.
16	Aerobics	5 mi.	8 mi.	5 mi.	Rest	4 mi.	12 mi.
17	Aerobics	4 mi.	6 mi.	4 mi.	Rest	4 mi.	8 mi.
18	Aerobics	3 mi.	4 mi.	Rest	Rest	1–3 mi.	MARATHON

start at a higher level than those done by beginners. In the first intermediate program, long runs start at 8 miles and progress 1 mile per week to 20 miles in the 13th week. This results in two 20-milers leading up to the marathon. The second intermediate program starts at 10 miles and has three 20-milers. The lengths of the midweek tempo runs also differ slightly. Important in each is the fact that every third week features a step-back for recovery.

The total weekly mileage progresses similarly, with approximately 60 percent of the mileage occurring at midweek and the rest in the weekend long run.

Expert Schedule

This is high-performance territory. In skiing terms it's black diamond: a steep mogul run. The expert schedule should be used only by very experienced marathoners, those who are seeking personal bests and are very familiar with the training necessary for peak performance. This 18-week training schedule takes a jump beyond that suggested for intermediate runners by adding speedwork. The week's work divides into six phases.

Base (Monday, Wednesday). These are the recovery days for expert runners and consist of short workouts run at easy pace. The primary focus for these easy days is to recover for the harder runs that are scheduled other days.

Tempo (Tuesday). Begin and end the tempo run at easy pace with 20 to 40 minutes of faster running in the middle at crisp pace. At the peak of the workout, you should be running close to 10-K pace.

Speedwork (Thursday). This consists of repeat runs of 800 to 1600 meters done at marathon pace on a track or measured straightaway. Rest between repeats by walking and/or jogging for 3 to 5 minutes. (Speedwork at shorter distances and at faster paces is best reserved for outside the marathon buildup period.)

Pace (Saturday). Begin and finish easy, but otherwise run near the pace at which you plan to race the marathon. Save some energy for Sunday's long run.

Distance (Sunday). A long run for expert runners is scheduled for Sunday but can be done any day. Run 1 to 2 minutes slower than the pace at which you plan to run the marathon. Just cover the distance; don't worry about time.

Rest. A rest day is included on Friday to help relieve the stress from accumulated mileage. Runners should program other days of complete rest when necessary.

Key to the expert program is the addition of speedwork on Thursday. A tempo run on Tuesday is also slightly faster than that done by intermediate runners. And there is more midweek running at marathon pace. But don't make the mistake of doing your long run too

Expert

WEEK	MON.	TUES.	WED.	THURS.	FRI.	SAT.	SUN.
1	3 mi.	5 mi.	3 mi.	4 x 800	Rest	5 mi.	10 mi.
2	3 mi.	5 mi.	3 mi.	5 x 800	Rest	5 mi.	11 mi.
3	3 mi.	4 mi.	3 mi.	6 x 800	Rest	6 mi.	8 mi.
4	3 mi.	6 mi.	3 mi.	4 x 1200	Rest	6 mi.	13 mi.
5	3 mi.	7 mi.	3 mi.	4 x 800	Rest	7 mi.	14 mi.
6	3 mi.	5 mi.	3 mi.	5 x 1200	Rest	7 mi.	10 mi.
7	3 mi.	8 mi.	3 mi.	5 x 800	Rest	8 mi.	16 mi.
8	4 mi.	8 mi.	4 mi.	6 x 1200	Rest	8 mi.	17 mi.
9	4 mi.	6 mi.	4 mi.	3 x 1600	Rest	9 mi.	12 mi.
10	4 mi.	9 mi.	4 mi.	6 x 800	Rest	9 mi.	19 mi.
11	4 mi.	10 mi.	4 mi.	4 x 1600	Rest	10 mi.	20 mi.
12	5 mi.	6 mi.	5 mi.	4 x 1200	Rest	6 mi.	12 mi.
13	5 mi.	10 mi.	5 mi.	5 x 1600	Rest	10 mi.	20 mi.
14	5 mi.	6 mi.	5 mi.	5 x 1200	Rest	6 mi.	12 mi.
15	5 mi.	10 mi.	5 mi.	6 x 1600	Rest	10 mi.	20 mi.
16	5 mi.	8 mi.	5 mi.	5 x 1200	Rest	4 mi.	12 mi.
17	4 mi.	6 mi.	4 mi.	4 x 800	Rest	4 mi.	8 mi.
18	3 mi.	4 mi.	3 mi.	Rest	Rest	1–3 mi.	MARATHON

fast. You do not want to detract from the hard workouts scheduled on other days. Running the weekend long run too fast is a sure route to overtraining and injury. And it's important to note that every third week features a step-back for recovery.

Total weekly mileage for expert runners is not much higher than for intermediate runners. If you feel you need additional mileage, increase the length of the runs on your easy days, but beware of overtraining. Twice-daily workouts are not recommended except for those runners with near-Olympian ambitions. Training at levels beyond those in this schedule probably should be attempted only by the most experienced runners and under the supervision of a knowledgeable coach.

10

MARATHON ELITE
BENJI DURDEN'S 84-WEEK PROGRAM

T his is the training program that caught the attention of my seatmates on the flight to Salt Lake City (mentioned in the introduction). They were interested in an article in an issue of *Runner's World* magazine, titled "The Path to Marathon Success."

The two executives spent most of their flight poring over the training schedules, analyzing each workout. The intensity of their interest was one reason that I decided to write this book.

The article was written by Benji Durden, a computer specialist from Boulder, Colorado. Durden has a marathon best of 2:09:58 (third at Boston in 1983) and was a member of the 1980 U.S. Olympic team. He also has experienced significant success coaching other athletes—everyone from Kim Jones (2:26:40) to recreational runners.

For an earlier *Runner's World* article, I had recruited Durden as one of three experts to advise a reader on how to train for a marathon. I liked Durden's schedule enough that I used it to train for my next marathon. The magazine's executive editor, Amby Burfoot, felt the same way and commissioned the article by Durden to expand on what he had said in my article.

But neither article did justice to the full program. There is never enough room in a monthly magazine, so we showed only 15 weeks. For this book, I asked Durden to design a marathon training program that lasted as long as he wanted. He offered this one, which lasts 84 weeks!

Not Your Average Program

The result might be described as "A Year and a Half in the Life of a Marathon Runner." This program is *not* for beginners. It is not for someone who began jogging last year and has reached the point where he has started to think, "Gee, it might be fun to run a marathon." No insult is intended, but this program is designed for athletes for whom running and racing have become a lifestyle. Durden's 84-week program includes two marathons among a total of 25 races. If you don't think he is serious about training, consider one workout from the 77th week: After doing a half-hour warmup, you run 5 × 800 and 5 × 400 on the track and conclude with a half-hour cooldown.

That's enough to scare almost anyone, but for someone who has been training for 77 weeks following Durden's advice, this workout is just part of a natural progression. In other words, if you can get to week 77, you can handle that one workout.

Actually, if you examine Durden's program you will discover that it is basically simple. It features a long run on the weekend and two midweek speed workouts. Everything else is easy jogging to recover for the next hard run. Here are the key elements.

Long run. Except when racing, Durden's athletes run long each weekend (Sunday). He prefers dictating long runs by minutes rather than miles, feeling that this takes the emphasis off how fast the miles are run. "Running too fast on the long workouts affects the quality of your speed workouts," Durden says. He recommends going 1 to 2 minutes per mile slower than your marathon pace. "Trust me on this," he says.

Speed training. Once a week (Tuesday), Durden's runners head for the hills—or to the track. He begins with a buildup of repeats on a hill with a 4 to 6 percent grade that takes about 90 seconds to run. (If you don't have a hill with that pitch or length, do the best you can.) Starting with three hill repeats, the runner builds to eight to nine repeats, then switches to the track to run 800 repeats on a similar buildup. The pace for the repeats should be hard, a near-maximum effort. Jog 400 meters between repeats. Warm up (wup) before and cool down (cdn) after the workout. For example, "20 wup/cdn" means a 20-minute warmup at easy pace before the repeats and a 20-minute similarly paced cooldown afterward.

Tempo run. Once a week (Thursday), Durden's runners do a tempo run—continuous runs (preferably on trails) that begin and end easy with fast running at varying speeds in the middle. The fast portions should be done at approximately the pace you can maintain for an hour (somewhat slower than 10-K race pace). "This should be a fast effort, but not exhausting," Durden writes. "If it's too fast, back off." Here is how you would run the workout labeled "18 wup/cdn, 2 (5 crisp/3 easy)" in week 7. (The "2" indicates that you run what is listed in the parentheses twice, with the exception of the final easy portion, which is part of the cooldown. Complicated? Sure, but you'll soon get used to the pattern.)

- 18 wup: 18-minute warmup at easy pace
- 5 crisp: 5 minutes at crisp pace
- 3 easy: 3 minutes at easy pace
- 5 crisp: 5 minutes at crisp pace
- 18 cdn: 18-minute cooldown at easy pace

Rest. Durden believes so strongly in the value of rest that he listed it first in his *Runner's World* article. "Rest, or easy days, are the most overlooked part of many programs," he writes. He schedules four days (Monday, Wednesday, Friday, and Saturday) for mostly half-hour jogs.

Maximum training. After the first marathon (week 43), Durden asks you to work even harder to prepare for the second one. He adds a second easy run to the long days. "I have a limit on how far I want anyone to run at one time," Durden explains, "but I want to increase the stress load. The goal is to increase the total amount of time you spend on your feet in one 12-hour period." The track workouts become more extensive, featuring distances other than the 800s that are used in the first buildup. Even the runs on easy days are somewhat longer. Training at this level will appeal to only the most dedicated runners.

Races. Durden believes that a certain amount of competition keeps runners "race sharp." He recommends racing every third or fourth week, but without putting any particular focus on these races (which substitute for the long runs in those weeks). Twice during the program (weeks 19 and 59), he schedules mini-peak races at near half-marathon distances. Before and after each, he adjusts the schedule to permit a short taper and recovery. Longer tapers and recoveries surround the marathons (weeks 43 and 84). In coaching athletes, even the elite, Durden strongly emphasizes the importance of rest during the week before races.

A year and a half is a long time to devote to any single training program, but if you are serious about achieving the "Marathon Success" that was guaranteed in the *Runner's World* article, you'll find that it's worth giving Durden's program a try. Even if you're not a marathoner, adapting a pattern similar to this schedule can make you a better runner.

There is an important reason that this type of program can have such significant benefits. For athletes who plan to make running a lifetime activity, training for any distance is something that needs to occupy more than the 8, 18, or even 84 weeks encompassed in any of the training programs outlined in this book. A commitment to lifetime running involves three phases: getting in shape, peaking for some special race, then backing down and resting before seeking a new peak. Durden's program demonstrates a workable pattern for doing this.

Benji Durden's Marathon Program

Week	Mon.	Tues.	Wed.	Thurs.	Fri.	Sat.	Sun.
1	30 jog	15 wup/cdn 3 hills hard	30 jog	15 wup/cdn 10 crisp	30 jog	30 jog	40 easy
2	30 jog	15 wup/cdn 4 hills hard	30 jog	15 wup/cdn 2 (5 crisp/ 3 easy)	30 jog	30 jog	1:00 easy
3	30 jog	16 wup/cdn 5 hills hard	30 jog	16 wup/cdn 12 crisp	30 jog	30 jog	1:10 easy
4	30 jog	15 wup/cdn 4 hills hard	30 jog	16 wup/cdn 10 crisp	30 jog	30 jog	**5-K— 10-K** RACE
5	30 jog	16 wup/cdn 5 hills hard	30 jog	17 wup/cdn 15 crisp	30 jog	30 jog	1:20 easy
6	30 jog	17 wup/cdn 6 hills hard	30 jog	17 wup/cdn 2 (8 crisp/ 4 easy)	30 jog	30 jog	1:45 easy
7	30 jog	18 wup/cdn 5 hills hard	30 jog	18 wup/cdn 2 (5 crisp/ 3 easy)	30 jog	30 jog	2:00 easy
8	30 jog	18 wup/cdn 6 hills hard	30 jog	18 wup/cdn 2 (10 crisp/ 5 easy)	30 jog	30 jog	**5-K— 10-K** RACE
9	30 jog	20 wup/cdn 7 hills hard	30 jog	20 wup/cdn 3 (7 crisp/ 4 easy)	30 jog	30 jog	2:10 easy
10	30 jog	22 wup/cdn 7 hills hard	30 jog	20 wup/cdn 4 (5 crisp/ 6 easy)	30 jog	30 jog	2:05 easy
11	30 jog	22 wup/cdn 7 hills hard	30 jog	22 wup/cdn 2 (12 crisp/ 6 easy)	30 jog	30 jog	2:30 easy
12	30 jog	22 wup/cdn 8 hills hard	30 jog	22 wup/cdn 3 (8 crisp/ 4 easy)	30 jog	30 jog	**8-K— 12-K** RACE

WEEK	MON.	TUES.	WED.	THURS.	FRI.	SAT.	SUN.
13	30 jog	24 wup/cdn 5 x 800 hard	30 jog	24 wup/cdn 5 (6 crisp/ 3 easy)	30 jog	30 jog	2:20 easy
14	30 jog	24 wup/cdn 5 x 800 hard	30 jog	24 wup/cdn 5 (5 crisp/ 3 easy)	30 jog	30 jog	2:40 easy
15	30 jog	26 wup/cdn 6 x 800 hard	30 jog	26 wup/cdn 2 (14 crisp/ 7 easy)	30 jog	30 jog	2:30 easy
16	30 jog	26 wup/cdn 5 x 800 hard	30 jog	26 wup/cdn 3 (9 crisp/ 5 easy)	30 jog	30 jog	10-K— 15-K RACE
17	30 jog	28 wup/cdn 6 x 800 hard	30 jog	28 wup/cdn 4 (7 crisp/ 4 easy)	30 jog	30 jog	2:25 easy
18	35 jog	45 easy	1:20 easy	35 jog	30 jog	30 jog	2:00 easy
19	35 jog	35 easy	30 jog	1:20 easy	30 jog	30 jog	15-K— 21-K RACE
20	35 jog	18 wup/cdn 5 hills hard	30 jog	16 wup/cdn 12 crisp	30 jog	30 jog	2:00 easy
21	35 jog	18 wup/cdn 6 hills hard	30 jog	16 wup/cdn 2 (6 crisp/ 3 easy)	30 jog	30 jog	2:25 easy
22	35 jog	19 wup/cdn 7 hills hard	30 jog	17 wup/cdn 15 crisp	30 jog	30 jog	2:20 easy
23	35 jog	19 wup/cdn 6 hills hard	30 jog	17 wup/cdn 2 (8 crisp/ 4 easy)	30 jog	30 jog	8-K— 12-K RACE
24	35 jog	20 wup/cdn 7 hills hard	30 jog	18 wup/cdn 3 (5 crisp/ 3 easy)	30 jog	30 jog	2:35 easy

(continued)

Benji Durden's Marathon Program—Continued

WEEK	MON.	TUES.	WED.	THURS.	FRI.	SAT.	SUN.
25	35 jog	20 wup/cdn 8 hills hard	30 jog	18 wup/cdn 2 (10 crisp/ 5 easy)	30 jog	30 jog	3:00 easy
26	35 jog	22 wup/cdn 7 hills hard	30 jog	20 wup/cdn 3 (7 crisp/ 4 easy)	30 jog	30 jog	2:20 easy
27	35 jog	22 wup/cdn 8 hills hard	30 jog	20 wup/cdn 4 (5 crisp/ 3 easy)	30 jog	30 jog	10-K— 10-MI. RACE
28	35 jog	24 wup/cdn 9 hills hard	30 jog	22 wup/cdn 2 (12 crisp/ 6 easy)	30 jog	30 jog	2:40 easy
29	35 jog	24 wup/cdn 8 hills hard	35 jog	22 wup/cdn 3 (8 crisp/ 4 easy)	30 jog	30 jog	3:10 easy
30	35 jog	26 wup/cdn 4 x 800 hard	35 jog	24 wup/cdn 4 (6 crisp/ 3 easy)	30 jog	30 jog	2:20 easy
31	35 jog	26 wup/cdn 5 x 800 hard	35 jog	24 wup/cdn 5 (5 crisp/ 2 easy)	30 jog	30 jog	21-K— 35-K RACE
32	35 jog	28 wup/cdn 6 x 800 hard	35 jog	26 wup/cdn 2 (14 crisp/ 7 easy)	30 jog	30 jog	2:45 easy
33	35 jog	28 wup/cdn 5 x 800 hard	35 jog	26 wup/cdn 3 (9 crisp/ 5 easy)	30 jog	30 jog	3:25 easy
34	35 jog	28 wup/cdn 6 x 800 hard	35 jog	28 wup/cdn 4 (7 crisp/ 4 easy)	30 jog	30 jog	5-K— 10-K RACE
35	35 jog	28 wup/cdn 7 x 800 hard	35 jog	28 wup/cdn 2 (15 crisp/ 8 easy)	30 jog	30 jog	2:50 easy
36	35 jog	30 wup/cdn 6 x 800 hard	35 jog	28 wup/cdn 3 (10 crisp/ 5 easy)	30 jog	30 jog	3:30 easy
37	35 jog	30 wup/cdn 7 x 800 hard	35 jog	30 wup/cdn 4 (8 crisp/ 4 easy)	30 jog	30 jog	5-K— 10-K RACE

WEEK	MON.	TUES.	WED.	THURS.	FRI.	SAT.	SUN.
38	35 jog	30 wup/cdn 8 x 800 hard	35 jog	30 wup/cdn 5 (6 crisp/ 3 easy)	30 jog	30 jog	2:20 easy
39	35 jog	32 wup/cdn 7 x 800 hard	35 jog	32 wup/cdn 6 (5 crisp/ 3 easy)	30 jog	30 jog	**15-K— 21-K** RACE
40	35 jog	32 wup/cdn 8 x 800 hard	35 jog	32 wup/cdn 3 (11 crisp/ 6 easy)	30 jog	30 jog	3:00 easy
41	35 jog	32 wup/cdn 9 x 800 hard	35 jog	32 wup/cdn 4 (9 crisp/ 5 easy)	30 jog	30 jog	**5-K— 10-K** RACE
42	35 jog	45 jog	1:30 easy	30 jog	30 jog	25 jog	2:00 easy
43	Rest	Rest	Rest	Rest	30 jog	30 jog	**MARATHON**
44	40 jog	40 jog	35 jog	40 jog	35 jog	35 jog	1:10 easy
45	40 jog	20 wup/cdn 5 hills hard	35 jog	18 wup/cdn 2 (10 crisp/ 5 easy)	35 jog	35 jog	A.M.: 1:20 easy P.M.: 30 jog
46	40 jog	20 wup/cdn 6 hills hard	35 jog	18 wup/cdn 3 (7 crisp/ 4 easy)	35 jog	35 jog	A.M.: 1:45 easy P.M.: 30 jog
47	40 jog	22 wup/cdn 7 hills hard	35 jog	18 wup/cdn 2 (5 crisp/ 2 easy)	35 jog	35 jog	A.M.: 2:00 easy P.M.: 30 jog
48	40 jog	22 wup/cdn 6 hills hard	35 jog	18 wup/cdn 4 (5 crisp/ 3 easy)	35 jog	35 jog	**5-K— 10-K** RACE
49	40 jog	24 wup/cdn 7 hills hard	35 jog	20 wup/cdn 2 (12 crisp/ 6 easy)	35 jog	35 jog	A.M.: 2:10 easy P.M.: 30 jog
50	40 jog	24 wup/cdn 8 hills hard	35 jog	20 wup/cdn 3 (8 crisp/ 4 easy)	35 jog	35 jog	A.M.: 2:05 easy P.M.: 30 jog

(continued)

WEEK	MON.	TUES.	WED.	THURS.	FRI.	SAT.	SUN.
51	40 jog	26 wup/cdn 7 x 800 hard	35 jog	18 wup/cdn 2 (5 crisp/ 2 easy)	35 jog	35 jog	A.M.: 2:30 easy P.M.: 30 jog
52	40 jog	26 wup/cdn 8 hills hard	35 jog	22 wup/cdn 4 (6 crisp/ 3 easy)	35 jog	35 jog	**5-K— 12-K** RACE
53	40 jog	28 wup/cdn 9 hills hard	35 jog	22 wup/cdn 5 (5 crisp/ 3 easy)	35 jog	35 jog	A.M.: 2:20 easy P.M.: 30 jog
54	40 jog	28 wup/cdn 3 x 800 hard	35 jog	24 wup/cdn 2 (14 crisp/ 7 easy)	35 jog	35 jog	A.M.: 2:40 easy P.M.: 30 jog
55	40 jog	28 wup/cdn 4 x 800 hard	35 jog	20 wup/cdn 2 (5 crisp/ 2 easy)	35 jog	35 jog	A.M.: 2:30 easy P.M.: 30 jog
56	40 jog	28 wup/cdn 5 x 800 hard	35 jog	24 wup/cdn 3 (9 crisp/ 5 easy)	35 jog	35 jog	**10-K— 15-K** RACE
57	40 jog	28 wup/cdn 3 x 800 hard	35 jog	28 wup/cdn 4 (7 crisp/ 4 easy)	35 jog	35 jog	A.M.: 2:25 easy P.M.: 30 jog
58	40 jog	28 wup/cdn 6 x 400 hard	35 jog	1:10 easy	35 jog	35 jog	A.M.: 2:00 easy P.M.: 30 jog
59	40 jog	40 jog	40 jog	25 wup/cdn 6 hills hard	35 jog	35 jog	**15-K— 21-K** RACE
60	40 jog	25 wup/cdn 7 hills hard	40 jog	24 wup/cdn 2 (14 crisp/ 7 easy)	35 jog	35 jog	A.M.: 2:30 easy P.M.: 30 jog
61	40 jog	27 wup/cdn 6 hills hard	40 jog	24 wup/cdn 3 (9 crisp/ 5 easy)	35 jog	35 jog	A.M.: 2:20 easy P.M.: 30 jog
62	40 jog	27 wup/cdn 7 hills hard	40 jog	22 wup/cdn 4 (7 crisp/ 4 easy)	35 jog	35 jog	**5-K— 10-K** RACE
63	40 jog	27 wup/cdn 8 hills hard	40 jog	22 wup/cdn 2 (15 crisp/ 8 easy)	35 jog	35 jog	A.M.: 2:45 easy P.M.: 30 jog

Benji Durden's Marathon Program—Continued

Week	Mon.	Tues.	Wed.	Thurs.	Fri.	Sat.	Sun.
64	40 jog	30 wup/cdn 7 hills hard	40 jog	20 wup/cdn 2 (5 crisp/ 2 easy)	35 jog	35 jog	A.M.: 2:25 easy P.M.: 30 jog
65	40 jog	30 wup/cdn 8 hills hard	40 jog	26 wup/cdn 3 (10 crisp/ 5 easy)	35 jog	35 jog	**8-K— 12-K** RACE
66	40 jog	30 wup/cdn 9 hills hard	40 jog	26 wup/cdn 4 (8 crisp/ 3 easy)	35 jog	35 jog	A.M.: 3:00 easy P.M.: 30 jog
67	40 jog	28 wup/cdn 4 x 800 hard 4 x 400 hard	40 jog	20 wup/cdn 2 (5 crisp/ 2 easy)	35 jog	35 jog	A.M.: 2:30 easy P.M.: 30 jog
68	40 jog	28 wup/cdn 5 x 800 hard 5 x 400 hard	40 jog	26 wup/cdn 5 (6 crisp/ 2 easy)	35 jog	35 jog	**5-K— 10-K** RACE
69	40 jog	28 wup/cdn 6 x 800 hard 6 x 400 hard	40 jog	26 wup/cdn 6 (5 crisp/ 2 easy)	35 jog	35 jog	A.M.: 3:10 easy P.M.: 30 jog
70	40 jog	28 wup/cdn 5 x 800 hard 5 x 400 hard	40 jog	20 wup/cdn 2 (5 crisp/ 2 easy)	35 jog	35 jog	A.M.: 2:30 easy P.M.: 30 jog
71	40 jog	27 wup/cdn 6 x 800 hard 6 x 400 hard	40 jog	28 wup/cdn 20 crisp/ 6 easy/ 20 crisp	35 jog	35 jog	**10-K— 10-MI.** RACE
72	40 jog	27 wup/cdn 4 x 1000 hard 4 x 600 hard	40 jog	28 wup/cdn 3 (12 crisp/ 4 easy)	35 jog	35 jog	A.M.: 3:30 easy P.M.: 30 jog
73	40 jog	27 wup/cdn 7 hills hard	40 jog	20 wup/cdn 2 (5 crisp/ 2 easy)	35 jog	35 jog	A.M.: 2:30 easy P.M.: 30 jog
74	40 jog	30 wup/cdn 8 hills hard	40 jog	28 wup/cdn 4 (9 crisp/ 3 easy)	35 jog	35 jog	**5-K— 10-K** RACE
75	40 jog	30 wup/cdn 9 hills hard	40 jog	20 wup/cdn 2 (5 crisp/ 2 easy)	35 jog	35 jog	A.M.: 3:30 easy P.M.: 30 jog

(continued)

Benji Durden's Marathon Program—Continued

Week	Mon.	Tues.	Wed.	Thurs.	Fri	Sat.	Sun.
76	40 jog	30 wup/cdn 10 x 400 hard	40 jog	20 wup/cdn 2 (5 crisp/ 2 easy)	35 jog	35 jog	A.M.: 2:00 easy P.M.: 30 jog
77	40 jog	40 jog	40 jog	30 wup/cdn 5 x 800 5 x 400	35 jog	35 jog	21-K— 30-K RACE
78	40 jog	30 wup/cdn 5 x 1000 hard 5 x 400 hard	40 jog	30 wup/cdn 4 (8 crisp/ 4 easy)	35 jog	35 jog	A.M.: 2:30 easy P.M.: 30 jog
79	40 jog	30 wup/cdn 6 x 800 hard 6 x 400 hard	40 jog	30 wup/cdn 5 (6 crisp/ 3 easy)	35 jog	35 jog	A.M.: 3:15 easy P.M.: 30 jog
80	40 jog	30 wup/cdn 12 x 400 hard	40 jog	20 wup/cdn 2 (5 crisp/ 2 easy)	35 jog	35 jog	A.M.: 2:40 easy P.M.: 30 jog
81	40 jog	25 wup/cdn 5 x 800 hard 5 x 400 hard 5 x 200 hard	40 jog	20 wup/cdn 6 (5 crisp/ 2 easy)	35 jog	35 jog	5-K— 10-MI. RACE
82	40 jog	20 wup/cdn 6 x 1000 hard 6 x 400 hard	40 jog	20 wup/cdn 3 (5 crisp/ 3 easy)	35 jog	35 jog	A.M.: 2:20 easy P.M.: 30 jog
83	40 jog	45 jog	1:30 easy	30 jog	30 jog	25 jog	A.M.: 2:00 easy
84	Rest	Rest	Rest	Rest	30 jog	30 jog	MARATHON

11

MULTIPLE MARATHONS
BEN MOORE'S REPEAT
AND THREEPEAT PROGRAM

In 1978, at the age of 53, Ben Moore, a former Marine Corps officer living in Annapolis, Maryland, ran his first marathon, a 4:30 at the Shamrock Marathon in Virginia Beach, Virginia. Soon after, he ran the Marine Corps Marathon and then three other marathons. That inspired his wife, Betty, to do the same.

"I told Betty that it was absolutely essential that she do the long runs," Moore recalls. "By that time I had five marathons under my belt, I naturally figured that I was eminently qualified to offer expert advice. I designed a training schedule featuring long runs on Saturdays and promised to help train her. It was the beginning of the running boom. Word spread in our neighborhood, and before I knew it, I had 18 women training for the 1980 Marine Corps Marathon."

They all trained at the same pace. If one person stopped for a drink, everyone stopped. If one had to go to the bathroom, everyone waited. Another runner named Bucky Cadell worked with Moore.

Moore would run at the front, with Cadell at the back to make sure that nobody was dropped. A member of the group purchased T-shirts for everyone to wear in the race, identifying them as "Moore's Marines." As in training, they ran together for 26 miles 385 yards, finishing under 4:30.

Moore looks back nostalgically on that first training group. "They were unique in that nobody had run before. They were all first-timers, starting at the same level. Tremendous *esprit* developed. You could never entirely recapture that, because now our marathon training groups are a blend of beginners and veterans. It's still exciting for everyone involved, but it's not quite the same."

In their 18th year in 1997, Moore's Marines are now affiliated with the Annapolis Striders, a local running group. As many as 100 runners enroll each July to follow a 14-week program that culminates in the Marine Corps Marathon, which is usually held the last weekend in October. Moore's Marines assemble each Saturday on Defense Highway and run an out-and-back route along that road, covering distances from 10 to 22 miles. On Sundays, some of the group meets again with the Striders at the city docks for a 10-mile run through the Naval Academy grounds.

Although the focus for the training program is the Marine Corps Marathon, Moore trains many in the group to run multiple marathons, and they go on to do the Memphis Marathon in December and/or the Disney World Marathon in January. "There are so many fine marathons," Moore says, "it's a shame to limit yourself to one a year."

Moore comes by his work ethic naturally. Born in 1925 in Grenada, Mississippi, he played halfback in football and ran the 220-yard low hurdles in track at the Naval Academy. "At 5 feet 8 inches and 165 pounds, I was probably the smallest person on the football team," he recalls. As a career Marine, Moore served in Korea and Vietnam and also coached football and track at the U.S. Marine Corps Base in Quantico, Virginia. Olympians on the Quantico track team included marathoner Alex Breckenridge, miler Pete Close, javelin thrower Al Cantello, and pole vaulter John Uelses. One speedy athlete from Philadelphia tried out for football at Quantico but failed (Moore claims) because "his legs were too skinny." The athlete achieved more success in track: high jumping, long jumping, and running relays. Later, he became an actor on television; his name is Bill Cosby. Moore also helped coach Roger Staubach on the plebe (freshman) football team at the Naval Academy.

Moore retired from the Marine Corps in 1969. "I had never done any distance running before, only what the Marine Corps required. But once out of the service, I began to work out at the field house, playing basketball and squash and eventually doing some road running." The next step was the marathon and the founding of Moore's Marines.

When One Is Not Enough

Moore's marathon training program is simple and basic and resembles many programs used by successful groups that are training marathoners in other cities. As with any marathon training program, you need a base level of fitness before starting. Moore's program involves a Saturday long run that gets progressively longer over a period of 14 weeks and an optional Sunday run of medium distance, usually 10 miles. The long run is done slower than marathon race pace; the medium run is done at race pace.

Once runners progress past 16 miles on their long runs, Moore recommends that if they run on Sunday, they do so at a much slower (jog) pace to avoid overtraining. Workouts on Monday through Thursday vary between hard (15 to 30 seconds faster than race pace) and easy (race pace). In keeping with the Universal Pace Chart (see page 9) in this book, Moore's hard pace is defined as medium (75 to 80 percent of maximum), his easy pace remains easy (65 to 75 percent), and his long-run pace is a jog (50 to 65 percent). Friday is a day of rest. In the peak week, Moore's Marines cover more than 50 miles.

Moore also suggests that on rest or optional days, runners do some cross-training such as swimming, bicycling, yoga, dancing, or stretching. He recommends adding strength training to the hard days (Tuesday and Thursday) but cautions, "If you need more rest, take it." On several days, he suggests that runners concentrate on "negative splits," running the second half of their workout faster than the first. "Runners need to adjust the plan to meet their needs and goals," he explains. "Beginning marathoners, obviously, should train more cautiously than more experienced runners."

Moore's Basic Program

WEEK	MON.	TUES.	WED.	THURS.	FRI.	SAT.	SUN.
1	5 mi. easy	5 mi. medium	5 mi. easy	5 mi. medium	Rest	10 mi. jog	10 mi. easy
2	5 mi. easy	5 mi. medium	5 mi. easy	5 mi. medium	Rest	12 mi. jog	10 mi. easy
3	5 mi. easy	5 mi. medium	5 mi. easy	5 mi. medium	Rest	14 mi. jog	10 mi. easy
4	6 mi. easy	6 mi. medium	6 mi. easy	6 mi. medium	Rest	12 mi. jog	10 mi. easy
5	6 mi. easy	6 mi. medium	6 mi. easy	6 mi. medium	Rest	14 mi. jog	10 mi. easy
6	6 mi. easy	6 mi. medium	6 mi. easy	6 mi. medium	Rest	Rest	**10-MI. RACE**
7	6 mi. easy	6 mi. medium	6 mi. easy	6 mi. medium	Rest	16 mi. jog	10 mi. jog
8	6 mi. easy	6 mi. medium	6 mi. easy	6 mi. medium	Rest	18 mi. jog	10 mi. jog
9	7 mi. easy	7 mi. medium	7 mi. easy	7 mi. medium	Rest	16 mi. jog	10 mi. jog
10	7 mi. easy	7 mi. medium	7 mi. easy	7 mi. medium	Rest	18 mi. jog	10 mi. jog
11	7 mi. easy	7 mi. medium	7 mi. easy	7 mi. medium	Rest	16 mi. jog	10 mi. jog
12	7 mi. easy	7 mi. medium	7 mi. easy	7 mi. medium	Rest	20 mi. jog	10 mi. jog
13	6 mi. easy	8 mi. medium	8 mi. easy	8 mi. medium	Rest	12 mi. jog	Rest
14	8 mi. easy	8 mi. easy	8 mi. easy	8 mi. easy	Rest	Rest	**FIRST MARATHON**

In Moore's basic program leading to the Marine Corps Marathon, on the opposite page, the 10-mile race appears in the sixth week, because that is the usual date of the Annapolis 10-Miler. Runners in other areas who are training for other marathons could insert a race of any distance from 10-K to a half-marathon at about this point in their

Four Weeks between Marathons

WEEK	MON.	TUES.	WED.	THURS.	FRI.	SAT.	SUN.
15	2 mi. easy	4 mi. easy	4 mi. easy	6 mi. medium	Rest	12 mi. jog	10 mi. jog
16	6 mi. easy	7 mi. medium	6 mi. easy	7 mi. medium	Rest	16 mi. jog	10 mi. jog
17	7 mi. easy	8 mi. medium	7 mi. easy	8 mi. medium	Rest	18 mi. jog	6 mi. jog
18	8 mi. easy	6 mi. medium	8 mi. easy	6 mi. medium	Rest	Rest	SECOND MARATHON

Six Weeks between Marathons

WEEK	MON.	TUES.	WED.	THURS.	FRI.	SAT.	SUN.
15	2 mi. easy	4 mi. easy	4 mi. easy	6 mi. medium	Rest	12 mi. jog	10 mi. jog
16	6 mi. easy	7 mi. medium	6 mi. easy	7 mi. medium	Rest	16 mi. jog	10 mi. jog
17	7 mi. easy	8 mi. medium	7 mi. easy	8 mi. medium	Rest	18 mi. jog	6 mi. jog
18	8 mi. easy	9 mi. medium	8 mi. easy	9 mi. medium	Rest	20 mi. jog	4 mi. jog
19	9 mi. easy	10 mi. medium	9 mi. easy	10 mi. medium	Rest	16 mi. jog	Rest
20	10 mi. easy	8 mi. medium	6 mi. easy	4 mi. easy	Rest	Rest	SECOND MARATHON

training. Moore considers an occasional race important to test conditioning.

In setting up his program so that runners can continue past this first marathon to run a second or even a third, Moore goes beyond the point where most other training programs stop. He advises that multiple marathoners program one easy week after their marathon efforts. Depending on how you feel, this might mean substituting walking for running. The final week before the next marathon is a tapering period to gather strength. In between those two rest weeks, runners can resume their regular training patterns. With only four weeks between marathons, Moore suggests running the first marathon at a slower pace, using it as a training run for the second.

Eight Weeks between Marathons

WEEK	MON.	TUES.	WED.	THURS.	FRI.	SAT.	SUN.
15	2 mi. easy	4 mi. easy	4 mi. easy	6 mi. medium	Rest	12 mi. jog	10 mi. jog
16	8 mi. easy	7 mi. medium	8 mi. easy	6 mi. medium	Rest	14 mi. jog	10 mi. jog
17	8 mi. easy	7 mi. medium	8 mi. easy	7 mi. medium	Rest	16 mi. jog	10 mi. jog
18	9 mi. easy	8 mi. medium	9 mi. easy	7 mi. medium	Rest	18 mi. jog	6 mi. jog
19	9 mi. easy	8 mi. medium	10 mi. easy	7 mi. medium	Rest	18 mi. jog	4 mi. jog
20	10 mi. easy	8 mi. medium	10 mi. easy	7 mi. medium	Rest	20 mi. jog	4 mi. jog
21	10 mi. easy	8 mi. medium	10 mi. easy	8 mi. medium	Rest	14 mi. jog	Rest
22	10 mi. easy	8 mi. easy	6 mi. easy	4 mi. easy	Rest	Rest	SECOND MARATHON

When you have six (or eight) weeks between marathons, Moore believes that you can begin to take the first one more seriously, racing both hard.

An extra 2 weeks between marathons allows a slightly different buildup. If you have 5, 7, or 9 weeks between marathons, you can adjust your schedule to fit. With more than 10 weeks between marathons, you may want to back up your training schedule to week 14 of the basic program and treat the next marathon as a single and separate race.

Running three marathons in a period of two months requires more adjustment. "This is truly pushing the edge of the envelope," Moore cautions. He suggests treating the first marathon as a training run and planning to run hard in the second marathon. And marathon number

Two More Marathons

WEEK	MON.	TUES.	WED.	THURS.	FRI.	SAT.	SUN.
15	2 mi. easy	4 mi. easy	4 mi. easy	6 mi. medium	Rest	12 mi. jog	10 mi. jog
16	6 mi. easy	7 mi. medium	6 mi. easy	7 mi. medium	Rest	16 mi. jog	10 mi. jog
17	7 mi. easy	8 mi. medium	7 mi. easy	8 mi. medium	Rest	18 mi. jog	6 mi. jog
18	8 mi. easy	6 mi. medium	8 mi. easy	6 mi. medium	Rest	Rest	**SECOND MARATHON**
19	2 mi. easy	4 mi. medium	4 mi. easy	6 mi. medium	Rest	12 mi. jog	10 mi. jog
20	6 mi. easy	7 mi. medium	6 mi. easy	7 mi. medium	Rest	16 mi. jog	10 mi. jog
21	7 mi. easy	8 mi. medium	7 mi. easy	8 mi. medium	Rest	18 mi. jog	6 mi. jog
22	10 mi. easy	8 mi. easy	6 mi. easy	4 mi. easy	Rest	Rest	**THIRD MARATHON**

three? Quoting a World War II song, Moore states, "You'll be coming home on a wing and a prayer."

Moore emphasizes that one way to achieve success in running multiple marathons is to not treat them equally. "Select one as the marathon in which you would like to achieve your peak performance. Then the marathon before or after that peak race can serve either as a training run, done at slower pace, or a run in which you race only to experience the sights and sounds around you. Every marathon you run does not have to be an all-out effort," he advises. Nevertheless, Moore discovered that despite racing hard at the Marine Corps Marathon in 1991, he ran even faster at the Memphis Marathon four weeks later, running a 3:47. "Sometimes, you surprise yourself," he says with a smile.

12

ULTRAS
GEORGE PARROTT'S
ULTRAMARATHON PROGRAM

On a Tuesday evening the Buffalo Chips gather in a shopping center parking lot on the east side of Sacramento, California. They are there for the club's weekly speed workout, organized by George Parrott, ultramarathoner, coach, and professor of psychology at California State University at Sacramento. Parrott offers few directions to the group, which soon numbers more than a hundred. The runners know why they've come and what to do. Soon they began to drift up onto the levee beside the American River—first the walkers, then the joggers, and eventually those who go still faster. As the workout continues, some begin doing a series of fast 1-mile repeats, designed by Parrott to get them in shape to run marathons—or ultramarathons, that netherworld beyond 26 miles 385 yards.

It is the contention of Coach Parrott that the Buffalo Chips is the strongest ultramarathon club in the United States, if not the world.

Despite what some might suspect, the Chips are not located in western New York. The club gets its name not from its city of origin but from the residue left on the ground after a buffalo moves on. (It began as a gag by club founders, but the name stuck.)

The Chips do run ultras more than most runners, and they also do better in them. The club includes in its ranks Tom Johnson (U.S. 100-K record-holder) and Rich Hanna (1994 and 1995 U.S. champion at that distance). Among the founders of the Chips, Abe Underwood ran 6:08 for 50 miles at age 40, and Paul Reese ran across the United States after passing age 70. "When I joined the club," Parrott smiles, "if you *didn't* run ultras, you were considered strange."

In 1978 Parrott ran his first ultra, the Lake Tahoe 72-Miler, which was founded by Reese. He finished with a time of 12:24. His next race was the Feather River 50-Mile, which he completed in 6:58. "I discovered that ultramarathons were survivable," he says. "Moreover, the training supported my particular running skills, which include a remarkable lack of speed." Skills or not, Parrott has run a 2:41 marathon and recently won a national 50-to-54 age-group title at 100-K (62.1 miles).

When coaching others, Parrott draws upon his own experience as a runner of limited ability who has achieved some degree of success. When members of the Buffalo Chips catch ultramarathon fever, he instructs them how to move beyond 26 miles 385 yards without compromising either their careers or their social lives. He also shows them how to avoid the injuries that so often accompany overtraining.

The 50-K

"The first step beyond the marathon," Parrott says, "is often 50 kilometers (31.07 miles), a standard race distance. For many, that's as far as they will venture into the ultramarathon world. Even if you're not racing that far, I regularly urge performance-oriented marathoners to complete 50-K runs during their buildup." Parrott believes that any well-trained marathoner can go that far. "Fifty kilometers is simply a marathon with a warmup."

Part of the secret of ultramarathon success is proper pacing. Parrott suggests that in their first 50-K, runners pass through 26 miles 385 yards with a split time 15 to 20 minutes slower than their marathon best (35 to 45 seconds per mile slower). They should then run the final 5 miles at a pace 60 seconds per mile slower. Thus, a 3:30 marathoner would finish a 50-K in about 4:30. Parrott believes that with more experience, they should be able to hit the marathon split within 10 minutes of their best effort and hold that pace to the finish. A 2:55 marathoner, for example, would finish in 3:35.

He also recommends that first-timers pick an ultramarathon that's run on either a point-to-point or large loop course rather than one with multiple laps. "Everyone experiences periods of mental and physical fatigue," he says. "You don't want to make it too easy to drop out." He suggests that, at least in your first ultra, you also avoid races that are made more difficult by terrain, high altitude, or the chance of extreme weather (heat or cold).

Key to Parrott's ultramarathon approach are rest days on Monday and Friday, before and after the long run that's done over the weekend. He refers to this as the sandwich approach, with the long run being the meat between two pieces of bread (the rest days). Tuesday is for speed training, such as the mile repeats. These are done at just faster than 10-K race pace. Wednesday and Thursday are for easy running at medium distances.

The "hardening" comes on the weekend with a Saturday tempo run, in which the middle miles are done at marathon race pace, and a long run on Sunday. Considering that the runner is preparing for an ultra, the total mileage (50 in the sample on page 88) is not exceptionally high. The pattern brings ultramarathon racing within the range of runners who have regular jobs and limited time to train.

Obviously, you would not do the week shown in the sample as the first week in your training program but rather toward the end of a steady buildup similar to those used to prepare runners for a standard marathon. This sample week is provided only as an example of the pattern used by Parrott.

Looking backward from the 50-K, Parrott would have his ultramarathoners training near the level shown in the sample eight weeks before the race. Then, as shown in the table on page 89, they would increase training distances for five weeks (1 through 5). The final four

Parrott's Sample Weekly Pattern

Day	Warmup/ Cooldown	Type of Training	Description	Pace	Daily Mileage
Mon.	—	Rest	—	—	0
Tues.	Warmup: 2 mi. jog Cooldown: 1 mi. jog	Speed training	3 x 1 mi. 2–3 min. jog between	Faster than 10-K pace (crisp)	6
Wed.	—	Steady run	8 mi.	Easy	8
Thurs.	—	Steady run	6 mi.	Easy	6
Fri.	—	Rest	—	—	0
Sat.	Warmup: 2 mi. jog Cooldown: 2 mi. jog (continuous)	Tempo run	3 mi. faster in middle	Marathon pace (medium)	7
Sun.	—	Long run	Walk during breaks	Easy	23
				Weekly Mileage	50

weeks (6 through 9) would be the taper, similar to those done in other training schedules. (He suggests running a 10-K race on the final weekend before the ultra as a final test of conditioning.)

"During long runs it is *very* important to drink regularly and take in further calories, using either sports drinks, energy gels, or foods rich in carbohydrates," Parrott comments. "This will help you to remain hydrated and preserve energy as much as possible, but it also teaches you how to take food and fluids during the race itself. You might be able to

Training for a 50-K

WEEK	MON.	TUES.	WED.	THURS.	FRI.	SAT.	SUN.	WEEKLY MILEAGE
1	Rest	3 x 1 mi. crisp	6 mi. easy	6 mi. easy	Rest	6 mi. tempo	20 mi. easy	50
2	Rest	3 x 1 mi. crisp	7 mi. easy	6 mi. easy	Rest	7 mi. tempo	23 mi. easy	50
3	Rest	3 x 1 mi. crisp	7 mi. easy	6 mi. easy	Rest	7 mi. tempo	24 mi. easy	51
4	Rest	4 x 1 mi. crisp	7 mi. easy	6 mi. easy	Rest	7 mi. tempo	25 mi. easy	53
5	Rest	4 x 1 mi. crisp	7 mi. easy	6 mi. easy	Rest	7 mi. tempo	26 mi. easy	54
6	Rest	5 x 1 mi. crisp	8 mi. easy	6 mi. easy	Rest	7 mi. tempo	20 mi. easy	50
7	Rest	4 x 1 mi. crisp	8 mi. easy	6 mi. easy	Rest	7 mi. tempo	14 mi. easy	43
8	Rest	3 x 1 mi. crisp	8 mi. easy	6 mi. easy	Rest	10-K RACE	5 mi. easy	34
9	Rest	3 x 1 mi. medium	8 mi. easy	3 mi. easy	2 mi. easy	Rest	50-K RACE	42

make it to the finish line in a marathon while skipping the water tables, but you won't in an ultra. Also important is finding out what products work for you. Everybody is different."

The 50-Mile

For experienced runners, moving from the marathon to the 50-K requires only a small leap of the imagination—a month or two added to the usual marathon training buildup. Moving from the 50-K to the 50-mile or 100-K requires considerably more *elan* on the part of the prospective ultramarathoner, but maybe not that much more talent or training. Parrott believes that runners of average ability can make this jump, without greatly increasing their training mileage, merely by tweaking the schedule and spending some extra time training on the weekends.

The weekend long run, of course, is the heart of all marathon training. For races above 50-K, Parrott prescribes long runs on both Saturday and Sunday.

"The basic Monday-through-Friday program remains the same," he says. "Some speed training is appropriate regardless of how long your race distance. National champions Tom Johnson and Rich Hanna regularly show up at club speedwork sessions to maintain their efficiency and sharpness."

Ultramarathoners training under Parrott's direction for 50-mile races continue their mileage progression by adding a second long run 10 weeks before the race (week 1 in the schedule on the opposite page). This is similar to the sandwich approach used for shorter distance training: two pieces of distance on Saturday and Sunday between two slices of rest on Friday and Monday.

Instead of thinking miles, Parrott suggests that ultramarathoners now think in terms of hours. They do Saturday and Sunday long runs for two weeks (1 and 2), and then do a recovery week with only one long run on the weekend, allowing the body to recuperate for the next thrust upward. (The estimated number of miles is listed in the table. It would vary from runner to runner, depending on how fast they ran those miles.)

For weeks 6 and 7 Parrott suggests that runners do the Saturday and Sunday runs over terrain similar to that of the planned event. (This is particularly important for trail ultras.) The last 2 hours on Sunday should be run at an increased heart rate level (80 percent) to simulate the stress of finishing strong.

On race day Parrott recommends recruiting as many support people as possible, both to provide food and fluids along the route and to run along in the closing miles in races that do not discourage pacing. When he ran his fastest 50-mile, two friends ran the final 10 miles with him, providing what he considered immeasurable support. "These longer distances are not easy, but with reasonable preparation, any marathoner can move up to the challenge of the ultra," he states.

Training for a 50-Mile or 100-K

Week	Mon.	Tues.	Wed.	Thurs.	Fri.	Sat.	Sun.	Weekly Mileage
1	Rest	4 x 1 mi. crisp	8 mi. easy	6 mi. easy	Rest	3 hr. easy	3–4 hr. easy	60
2	Rest	4 x 1 mi. crisp	8 mi. easy	6 mi. easy	Rest	3 hr. easy	3–4 hr. easy	60
3	Rest	4 x 1 mi. crisp	8 mi. easy	6 mi. easy	Rest	2 hr. easy	1 hr. easy	40
4	Rest	4 x 1 mi. crisp	8 mi. easy	6 mi. easy	Rest	3 hr. easy	3–4 hr. easy	60
5	Rest	4 x 1 mi. crisp	8 mi. easy	6 mi. easy	Rest	3 hr. easy	3–4 hr. easy	60
6	Rest	4 x 1 mi. crisp	8 mi. easy	6 mi. easy	Rest	4–5 hr. easy	3–3.5 hr. easy	75
7	Rest	4 x 1 mi. crisp	8 mi. easy	6 mi. easy	Rest	4–5 hr. easy	3–3.5 hr. easy	75
8	Rest	4 x 1 mi. crisp	8 mi. easy	6 mi. easy	Rest	1 hr. easy	1.5 hr. easy	35
9	Rest	3 x 1 mi. crisp	8 mi. easy	6 mi. easy	Rest	2 hr. easy	2 hr. medium	50
10	Rest	3 x 1 mi. crisp	8 mi. easy	6 mi. easy	Rest	1 hr. easy	1 hr. easy	30
11	Rest	3 x 1 mi. medium	4 mi. easy	3 mi. easy	2 mi. easy	Rest	50-MI. OR 100-K RACE	42

13

GIRLS' CROSS-COUNTRY
THE ELSTON HIGH SCHOOL
PROGRAM

In 1992 I served as head coach of the boys' and girls' cross-country teams at Elston High School in Michigan City, Indiana. It was my fourth year as coach. That year we took seven girls to the state championships in Indianapolis, six of whom were running their first year of high school cross-country. Two had never participated in any sport before. Our one veteran, a smooth-striding sophomore, was making her first trip to the state meet, as was her coach. We were definitely "New Kids on the Course." (I even had T-shirts made with that motto on the front.)

Nevertheless, we had one thing in our favor: talent. Combined with that were a desire to succeed and a basic love of running, some of which were acquired during a winning season. We were also a smart team, with an average 3.96 grade-point average.

At midseason, we sneaked into the rankings at number 19. We eventually rose to number 15, but at the state meet in Indianapolis, everyone on the team ran their best races of the year. We finished fifth.

The following is an account of the training and superb effort that led to the team's success during that season.

Summer Training

According to Indiana High School Athletic Association (IHSAA) rules, you can't hold "practice" during the summer. You can, however, get together for conditioning. If you're a football coach, your team can't throw the ball around or practice in pads, but they can lift weights and run drills. If you're a basketball coach, you can't play practice games, but the players can run and shoot. As a cross-country coach, I saw little distinction between what was practice and what was conditioning. We ran during the summer, which is what we did during the season as well. All other motivated coaches in Indiana, and in other states, operate the same way.

In starting to prepare for the season, I followed the advice taught to doctors in medical school: First, do no harm. I figured that if I could systematically undertrain my top girls, their natural abilities would emerge. Jack Daniels, Ph.D., the very successful track-and-field and cross-country coach from the State University of New York at Cortland, believes that 30 miles a week is plenty for young girls, with perhaps a maximum of 40. We trained well under Jack's red line: 25 weekly miles.

In past summers, when I scheduled daily practices, I never knew who might show. The only two days that everybody came were Tuesday and Thursday for the mandatory practices. On those mornings, we met on our home course. We began the summer by running 30 to 40 minutes, and by midsummer we had progressed to repeats on a 1-K loop.

Wednesday and Friday were optional. Most of us met in the early morning on a golf course for strides, bounding, and stretching. It was mainly play, hardly any mileage.

Each Monday, the team met at the beach in the evening for "water

Summer Training

Day	Time	Location	Effort	Workout
Mon.	30–60 min.	Beach	Easy	Stretching, playing
Tues.	30–40 min.	Trail	Easy	Cross-country run
Wed.	40 min.	Grass	Medium	Strides, bounding, stretching
Thurs.	30–40 min.	Trail	Easy	Cross-country run
Fri.	40 min.	Grass	Medium	Strides, bounding, stretching
Sat.	30–40 min.	Road	Easy	Optional run
Sun.	—	—	—	Rest

babies" with my assistant coach, Mary Taylor. It was Mary's "thing," so I never showed up. The girls went a couple of miles up the beach, stretched, swam, and ran back at a faster pace.

Midway through the summer, the team attended Coach Roy Benson's running camp in Asheville, North Carolina. (We took with us two talented eighth-grade girls, who would join the team the following year.) Afterward, we stepped up the pace of training back home. We attended one race as a group at the end of July: Steve's Run in Dowagiac, Michigan, a 10-K road and trail race.

Preseason Training

Official practice began three weeks before our first meet. This was our key period for getting people ready. We trained with higher intensity but didn't overlook recovery days. I don't believe in double workouts, except on occasion for veteran runners; the double workouts in the table on the opposite page were only for my better runners.

Along with offering team members a copy of the training program for that period, I included the following comments: "My assessment

Three Weeks in August

DAY/DATE	ACTIVITY	WORKOUT
MON./10	Organizational meeting	1600-meter time trial
TUES./11	Interval training, 600-meter trail	Multiple repeats
WED./12	Speedwork, golf course	Strides, bounding, stretching
THURS./13	Low-key race, trails	3–4 mi.
FRI./14	Hill training, sand dunes	Multiple uphill repeats
SAT./15	Long run, roads and trails	30–60 min. medium
SUN./16	Rest	—
MON./17	Interval training, 600-meter trail	Multiple repeats
TUES./18—A.M.	Speedwork (optional)	Strides, bounding, stretching
TUES./18—P.M.	Long run, roads and trails	Medium
WED./19	Fartlek, trails	Varied paces
THURS./20—A.M.	Speedwork (optional)	Strides, bounding, stretching
THURS./20—P.M.	Long run, roads and trails	Medium
FRI./21	Interval training, 600-meter trail	Multiple repeats
SAT./22	Long run, woods	30–60 min. easy
SUN./23	Rest	—
MON./24—A.M.	Speedwork (optional)	Strides, bounding, stretching
MON./24—P.M.	Interval training, 600-meter trail	Multiple repeats
TUES./25	Long run, roads and trails	30–45 min. medium
WED./26	Morning speedwork	Strides, bounding, stretching
THURS./27	First day of school	Repeats on a 1-K trail loop
FRI./28	Easy warmup	Jogging and stretching
SAT./29	Competition	INVITATIONAL MEET: 3000 METERS
SUN./30	Rest	—

of those who have trained through the summer is that we are in very good shape already. There's no reason for a crash training program. There's no reason to push hard every day. There's no reason to do extra workouts. Listen to the coaches. Rest is as important a component of a training program as speedwork. Don't go out and run 12 miles on Sunday thinking that it will get you in better shape; it may only get you injured and delay your progress.

"Newcomers (and those who trained less this summer) need to be cautious about matching stride with team leaders. Overtraining is the route to injury. We can only have a successful season if we stay healthy—and that means avoiding colds, a symptom of overtraining."

Looking back on that season, because of low-mileage training, we had almost zero injuries among our top runners. That was a major reason for our success. It was members of our second team who got hurt trying to catch up.

The first three weeks consisted of a variety of training. In listing repeats, such as those we did on a 600-meter loop in the woods, in the table, I don't list the number of repeats because it varied depending on each runner's level of ability. Usually, it was anywhere between 5 and 10 repeats; the number was based on the coaches' evaluation as they watched each runner and pulled them in and out of the pack as they ran the route through the woods. Similarly, on long runs we often would show trailing runners how to take shortcuts to cut mileage and catch the main group. As any coach will tell you, organizing workouts for runners of different levels of ability is the most difficult trick in achieving success for the overall program.

Midseason Training

During the regular season, there was little time to train. We participated in conference dual meets each Tuesday and invitational meets featuring large numbers of teams on Saturdays. Most of the members on our team were good students and wanted to maintain high grades. They also were involved in other activities, from student council to the drama club. I tried not to waste time in training, usually finishing each session within an hour. I felt that doing much more would be counterproductive. The following table shows our routine for a typical midseason week that included competition. It includes three hard days (two races with a workout featuring long repeats sandwiched between) and one medium day. Two days are very easy workouts before the races. The seventh day is rest.

A Typical Midseason Week		
DAY	**ACTIVITY**	**WORKOUT**
MON.	Easy workout	Warmup, strides, bounding
TUES.	Dual meet competition	**4000-METER RACE**
WED.	Tempo run, trails	Medium with fast middle
THURS.	Interval training, trails	4–5 x 1000 hard
FRI.	Easy workout	Warmup, strides, bounding
SAT.	Invitational competition	**4000-METER RACE**
SUN.	Rest	—

IHSAA regulations don't permit Sunday practices. I never ran with team members on Sunday, even meeting them "accidentally" as some coaches do. On a few occasions, I suggested to my top runners that they do an easy long run on Sunday. Most times, I preferred that they rest.

In my notes to the team, I discussed injuries: "Try to avoid them. Practice regularly. Don't overtrain. Don't run recklessly in workouts or in meets. Don't assume that an easy day allows you to play 2 hours of touch football afterward. Practice good nutrition: Eat a good breakfast. Avoid junk at lunch. Eat lots of fruits and veggies. Proper eating habits will help you maintain energy levels so you can perform well and avoid injuries."

Presectional

Following the last invitational, we had two weeks with no meets before the sectional, the first of the four-step qualification meets leading to the state championships. Next to preseason, I considered this

Two Weeks in October

Day/Date	Activity	Workout
Mon./5	Long run, trails	45 min. easy (recovery after Saturday meet)
Tues./6	Interval training, 600-meter trail	Multiple repeats
Wed./7	Easy speedwork	Strides, bounding, stretching
Thurs./8	Long repeats	3 x 1200 (sectional course)
Fri./9	Long run, trails	45 min. easy
Sat./10	Trail run	45 min. hilly course, hard
Sun./11	Rest	Optional run
Mon./12	Trail run	45 min. flat course hard
Tues./13	Long run, roads	60 min. easy
Wed./14	Short repeats	Canceled midworkout—rain
Thurs./15	Fartlek, trails	30 min. crisp to hard
Fri./16	Easy warmup	Strides, bounding, stretching
Sat./17	Sectional meet	**4000-METER RACE**

the key period for training. We followed the same hard/easy pattern, but without races in the way. It gave us time to heal and focus our minds.

Even though we made no attempt to peak, we took five of the top eight positions, setting a sectional record for a winning score. This was my first sectional victory in four years of coaching (although my boys' team had missed by only 7 points two years earlier), and it was definitely because of our team's talent.

Peak Training

We began tapering for the state championships the following Monday. To do this took a certain amount of chutzpah on the part of the coaches, since it assumed that we would qualify out of a loaded regional field with four ranked teams and an even tougher semi-state

The Final Three Weeks

Day	Activity	Workout
Mon.	Tempo run, trails	30–60 min. medium
Tues.	Long run, trails	30–40 min. easy
Wed.	Long repeats, trails	Week 1: 4 x 1000 hard Week 2: 4 x 700 hard Week 3: 4 x 400 hard
Thurs.	Morning warmup, grass	Easy strides
Fri.	Rest	—
Sat.	**4000-METER RACE**	Regional: 2nd place Semi-state: 4th place State: 5th place
Sun.	Rest	—

field that included seven ranked teams, six of which were ranked ahead of us. (Only four teams at each level qualified to advance to the next level.) I felt that we needed to make this assumption and take a risk if we wanted to do well at the state championships.

Going through the last three weeks, we maintained the intensity on hard days but cut distance. For instance, week 1's Monday run was 50 to 60 minutes over some good hills. For week 2, we ran 40 to 50 minutes over flat terrain. Week 3 was 30 to 40 minutes, but we stopped for a stretch break in the middle.

Each Thursday, we ran in the morning before school rather than in the afternoon. That was to give us a few more hours' rest between our pre-race workout and the race. The reason was psychological as well as physical.

The only change in schedule during the final week was to make Thursday our rest day (no running), then jog the course on Friday after arriving in Indianapolis. And the next day, we achieved a peak performance in the most important race of the year.

Going into the season, I had set three goals to be achieved over a three-year period: qualify for state, be competitive at state, and win state. I felt that, considering the competition in our area, the most difficult task would be to reach the first goal in the first year. After that, everything else should fall into place for the following two years, since the team was young, talented, and dedicated. Plus, the two eighth-graders that we had taken to camp (and who ran one-two at a major invitational for their grade level during the year) would be joining a veteran squad.

As it turned out, they achieved the first two goals in the first year, leaving the team with only one goal for the following two years. And they achieved it: The Elston High School girls' cross-country team won the state championship in both of those seasons.

14

SUMMER CROSS-COUNTRY
SAM BELL'S
TRAINING PROGRAM

Sam Bell has trained some of America's top distance runners, most recently Bob Kennedy, who set the American record for 5000 meters (12:58:21) during the summer of 1996 and placed sixth in that event at the Olympic Games. Other Bell Olympians include Morgan Groth (800, 1964), Jim Spivey (1500, 1984, 1992; 5000, 1996), Mark Deady (1500, 1988), and Terry Brahm (5000, 1988).

Bell was a multisport athlete at the small schools he attended in Nebraska. In high school he competed in football, basketball, baseball, and track and field, where his events were sprints, distance, pole vault, discus, high jump, and long jump. He qualified for the state championships in both the high jump and 880, but the height of his high school athletic career may have been a 99-yard touchdown run, the longest in the state that year.

After serving in the U.S. Navy during World War II, Bell continued as a half-miler at Doane College in Crete, Nebraska. Later, he coached at the University of California at Berkeley and Oregon State University in Corvallis, where his 1962 team won the NCAA cross-country championships. In 1969 he moved to Indiana University in Bloomington to serve as head coach for men's and women's cross-country and track and field. He has coached 19 NCAA and 269 Big Ten individual champions. His teams have won 26 Big Ten titles.

Bell believes that how runners train during the summer dictates their success in cross-country that fall as well as in track later in the year. Soon after members of his team return home after the spring quarter, he mails them a copy of summer workouts. Although these schedules may vary from year to year, the pattern remains the same.

Bell divides summer training into three periods, early summer, midsummer, and late summer. He divides workouts into three classes, called stress, semi-stress, and recovery. He also asks his runners to do one long run a week, which might fall into the semi-stress category.

Here is how Coach Bell explains the theory of stress versus semi-stress.

Stress. "A stress workout is one that takes the runner into a zone where work becomes anaerobic and somewhat duplicates what the body experiences while racing," he says. "Stress workouts prepare both the body and the mind to reach beyond where they normally want to go."

Semi-stress. "A semi-stress workout is by no means easy. You reach the discomfort zone but not the wall. These workouts in the early summer prepare runners for the stress workouts later on," Bell explains.

Recovery. "Recovery workouts are necessary because you can't run hard too often without risking staleness and injury," he says. "Yet you still need extra mileage to increase your aerobic base."

At the beginning of the summer, Bell's college runners do only two semi-stress workouts a week. As the summer continues and the time to return to school approaches, the training becomes progressively more difficult with the addition of another semi-stress day and the substitution of stress days for one or two of the semi-stress days.

Yet Bell avoids dictating workouts for any specific day. He provides examples of stress and semi-stress workouts and allows his athletes to choose from this menu to design their own training programs. Most veteran athletes at Indiana are familiar with the program after running under his guidance and that of women's coach Roseann Wilson.

Although Bell's schedule is designed to maintain and build the fitness of college-age athletes during the off-season, adult runners could also modify it for their own use in training for events as diverse as the 1500 meters or the marathon.

Early Summer

Most of Coach Bell's stress or semi-stress workouts feature changes of pace, following his belief that cross-country runners need to be prepared to change pace at any stage of the race. "If you're battling opponents, you can use pace changes and the terrain to defeat them. If the opponent initiates the pace change, you must be prepared to counter the move." Bell cites the 1992 NCAA cross-country championships, with Bob Kennedy battling Washington State's Joseph Kapkori. Midway through the 10,000-meter race, first Kapkori, then Kennedy, surged and countersurged in an attempt to break free. Kennedy pushed a short hill, then kept going. Kapkori looked over his shoul-

Early Summer Workouts		
WORKOUT	**TIME**	**PACE**
Semi-stress-A	35–50 min.	Medium
Semi-stress-B	10 min. 20–30 min. 5–10 min.	Crisp Medium Crisp
Semi-stress-C	10–15 min. 10–20 min. 10–15 min.	Medium Fartlek Medium
Recovery	25–35 min.	Easy
Long run	40–65 min.	Easy

der, more worried about runners behind than the runner in front. "The race was over," Bell recalls. "Kennedy won by 43 seconds."

An example of how Bell prescribes pace changes is apparent in the table below. In semi-stress workout B, the runner would begin with 10 minutes at a crisp pace, shift to 20 to 30 minutes at a medium pace (slightly slower), then finish with 5 to 10 more minutes at crisp pace.

Early Summer Schedule

WEEK	MON.	TUES.	WED.	THURS.	FRI.	SAT.	SUN.
1	Recovery	Semi-stress-A	Recovery	Recovery	Semi-stress-B	Recovery	40 min. easy
2	Recovery	Semi-stress-C	Recovery	Recovery	Semi-stress-A	Recovery	50 min. easy
3	Recovery	Semi-stress-B	Recovery	Recovery	Semi-stress-C	Recovery	65 min. easy

The first stage of summer training lasts a minimum of three weeks and could go for six weeks or more, depending upon the runner's level of conditioning and the amount of time available. (Runners who fail to qualify for the Big Ten championships in May begin their summer training early and may need to spend more time with this form of base training.)

Midsummer

At the appropriate time, runners shift into the second phase of their summer training by adding a single stress workout per week to go with the two semi-stress workouts.

Despite the difficulty of the training regimen, Bell considers recovery days as important as stress days. Also important is an awareness of when to deviate from the plan and seek extra rest. "It is important for runners to learn to read their bodies," he advises. "They must be able to recognize fatigue and determine when to push on and when the load must be lightened so the body can recover. There are times when you need to rest not just one day but two or three to avoid cumulative fatigue, which can lead to injury."

Midsummer Workouts

Workout	Time	Pace
Semi-stress-D	20 min. 15–25 x 100 10–15 min.	Medium Hard Medium
Stress-E	40–50 min.	Crisp
Stress-F	15–20 min. 15–20 min. 15–20 min.	Medium Fartlek Medium
Stress-G	35–40 min. 15–25 x 100	Crisp Hard
Stress-H	10 min. 10 min. 10 min. 10 min. 10 min.	Medium Crisp Medium Fartlek Medium
Recovery	25–40 min.	Easy
Long run	45–70 min.	Easy

Midsummer Schedule

Week	Mon.	Tues.	Wed.	Thurs.	Fri.	Sat.	Sun.
4	Recovery	Semi-stress-A	Recovery	Stress-E	Recovery	Semi-stress-D	45 min. easy
5	Recovery	Semi-stress-A	Recovery	Stress-F	Recovery	Semi-stress-D	50 min. easy
6	Recovery	Semi-stress-A	Recovery	Stress-G	Recovery	Semi-stress-D	55 min. easy
7	Recovery	Semi-stress-A	Recovery	Stress-H	Recovery	Semi-stress-D	60 min. easy
8	Recovery	Semi-stress-A	Recovery	Stress-E	Recovery	Semi-stress-D	65 min. easy
9	Recovery	Semi-stress-A	Recovery	Stress-F	Recovery	Semi-stress-D	70 min. easy

Late Summer

In the last month before Bell's runners return to campus, the intensity increases. Now there are two stress workouts combined with one semi-stress workout each week. Bell likes to see his runners progress from 30 to 40 to 50 to 70 miles a week during the summer. Depending on their abilities and levels of development, some runners will do more, and some will do less.

Late Summer Workouts

Workout	Time	Pace
Semi-stress-I	40–60 min.	Medium
Semi-stress-J	30–40 min. 20–30 x 100	Medium Hard
Semi-stress-K	20 min. 3000 meters	Medium Ins & outs (hard, easy, alternating paces)
Stress-L	10 min. 15–20 min. 10 min. 15–20 min. 10 min.	Medium Crisp Medium Crisp Medium
Stress-M	10 min. 5 min. 10 min. 15–20 min. 10–20 min.	Medium Fartlek Medium Fartlek Medium
Stress-N	10 min. 10 min. 5 min. 10–15 min. 10 min. 10–15 min.	Medium Crisp Hard Medium Fartlek Medium
Recovery	25–45 min.	Easy
Long run	45–75 min.	Easy

Late Summer Schedule

WEEK	MON.	TUES.	WED.	THURS.	FRI.	SAT.	SUN.
10	Recovery	Stress-L	Recovery	Semi-stress-I	Recovery	Stress- M	45 min. easy
11	Recovery	Stress-N	Recovery	Semi-stress-J	Semi-stress-A	Stress- L	60 min. easy
12	Recovery	Stress-M	Recovery	Semi-stress-K	Semi-stress-C	Stress- N	75 min. easy

The first cross-country meet is usually two to three weeks after runners return to campus and begin practice. Because runners who compete in cross-country, indoor track, and outdoor track may run in as many as two dozen meets during the school year, Bell does not encourage off-season racing. But he also doesn't prohibit it. To maintain motivation and test their fitness levels, Indiana runners jump into an occasional road race. Depending on how hard they run (to win or simply to collect a T-shirt), the race would substitute for either a stress or semi-stress workout. "Races are good if used to check progress in training," Bell says. "If runners are good enough to race at the national or international level, we encourage them to do so."

The final phase of the summer training schedule lasts three to four weeks, but it could be extended if more time is available.

Second Workouts

In addition to the workouts described above, veteran Indiana runners run a second time during the day. This second run lasts from 20 to 40 minutes and is run at what Bell describes as a gentle tempo ("easy," as defined in this book). He reasons that by training twice daily, runners can amass higher total mileage than they can with only one daily run. "It's easier to run 4 miles in the morning and 8 in the afternoon than 12 in one run," he says. The extra mileage allows his runners to build their aerobic base more efficiently. "This is true of a runner at any stage of development, from beginner to veteran," he says.

The table below illustrates how Bell's athletes progress during the summer from doing a single workout a day to training twice daily. In the first week, they would run a second time every other day and go from there. The times refer to how long his runners train; distance is not prescribed because runners vary in their abilities to run fast or slow. (Weather and terrain may also influence pace.)

Where there are two times listed, this indicates suggested workouts of varying lengths from day to day. For instance, runners do double workouts on six days in week 6. Three of the workouts are 20 minutes long and the other three are 25 minutes long. Most important, all of these runs are done at an easy pace.

Second Daily Run Schedule

Week	Frequency/week	Second Run Time	Intensity
1	3	20 min.	Easy
2	3	20 min.	Easy
3	4	20 min.	Easy
4	5	20 min.	Easy
5	6	20 min.	Easy
6	6	3 x 20 min. 3 x 25 min.	Easy
7	6	2 x 20 min. 4 x 25 min.	Easy
8	6	1 x 20 min. 5 x 25 min.	Easy
9	6	25 min.	Easy
10	3	30 min.	Easy
11	4	30 min.	Easy
12	5	30 min.	Easy

Eventually, of course, Bell's athletes run out of summer; but until then, the progression continues according to this general pattern until the runners are comfortable with doing 25- to 40-minute runs twice daily, six days a week.

Several days after the Indiana team members return to campus in the fall, they usually participate in a semi-competitive event that is called the Barbecue Run because after the race, they head to Coach Bell's house for just that. The men run the first half of the 8000-meter cross-country course at a medium pace, then finish hard. The women do the same over their 5000-meter course. And with that, the regular season begins.

15

TRACK

JOHN DAVIES'S PHASED PROGRAM

In 1961 at age 22, New Zealander John Davies competed in a handicap mile race against Murray Halberg, the Olympic 5000-meter champion from the previous year. Davies ran 4:15, which, with the aid of his handicap, allowed him to beat Halberg.

His effort impressed Arthur Lydiard, who, in addition to coaching Halberg, coached Olympic 800-meter champion Peter Snell. Lydiard invited Davies to train with his runners doing 22-milers on the hilly Owairaka course on the outskirts of Auckland, New Zealand. Within three years, Davies brought his mile time down to 3:56.8 and his 1500 time down to 3:39.6, which he ran to win the bronze medal, behind Snell, at the 1964 Olympics.

Davies hoped to move up to the 5000 for 1968, but a torn Achilles tendon ended his competitive career. He continues to run recreationally and serves as a coach and agent. His runners have included world record-holders Dick Quax and Anne Audain. He currently trains Toni Hodgkinson, who placed fifth in the 800 in the 1997 World Indoor Championships.

Davies suggests that while running times have improved significantly since the 1960s, training methods have not. He still believes in the theories pioneered by Lydiard. "Nobody has been able to improve on Lydiardism in the last 30 years," says Davies. "People always look for new ways to train. It disturbs me that coaches invent things just to put their own stamp on their training. Science has proved that there is no better way to train middle-distance runners than the way Arthur did 30 years ago. It's a very logical process."

Davies defines Lydiardism as a system that builds endurance, strength, speed, a high oxygen uptake, and a high lactate threshold in middle-distance runners. Based on their level of conditioning, athletes begin by doing long runs over a period of several months to develop an aerobic base, or endurance.

They then move into a second phase that includes hill training. "This is specific strength training where you do hill repeats and work your body weight against gravity," Davies explains. A third phase includes track training: large volumes of interval work, such as 20 $\times$ 200. "These interval workouts are done as continuous runs," he says, "with each repetition followed by an equal distance jogged." He notes that some runners mistake this for speed training, which Davies considers wrong. "A few coaches like to split these sessions into sets of, say, 5 $\times$ 400 with rests between sets. Again, it is an attempt to introduce speed into a workout where the true purpose is to develop lactate tolerance."

In the fourth and final phase, fine-tuning before the most important races, runners shift to true speedwork: short distances run flat out with long rests between—small numbers, like 3 $\times$ 200. "Arthur proved it worked with Snell and the others I trained with," insists Davies. "It still works today."

Phase Training

Perhaps the most unique contribution Lydiard made to distance training was what coaches today call periodization, doing different types of training at different times of the year. Davies describes this as phase training. "Phase training provides a psychological benefit as well as a physical benefit," he says. "You're less likely to burn out because, while you're training as hard as you can, you know that in a couple of weeks you'll move to a different phase and your training will change. You look forward to the next phase. You're not always on the roads. You're not always on the track. You're not always racing. Athletes today sometimes have difficulty figuring out when and how to peak. That was never a problem with Arthur's boys."

Even Davies's current star athlete, Hodgkinson, trains the way Lydiard trained everybody from half-milers to marathoners, although she does not quite do 22-mile runs. When Hodgkinson began running under Davies's supervision, she had to struggle to cover a 5-K in easy runs. By gradually building her endurance base over a period of four years, Davies built her long workouts up to a long run of 2 hours. During this period, her time in the 800 dropped from 2:07 to 1:58.

Davies believes that you can use phase training whether you are an 800-meter runner or a marathoner and whether your main interest as a competitive runner is track or cross-country or running the roads. Although he and Snell ran frequently with the marathon runners in Lydiard's stable of star athletes, when they moved into the third and fourth phases of their track training, their workouts shifted direction. The middle-distance runners ran shorter (and faster) repeats than those competing at longer distances.

The following programs detail how Davies coaches runners preparing for the traditional track middle distances (800 and 1500 meters). Davies's phased program would begin after a season of cross-country training and racing.

Phase 1: Endurance

The object of this first, endurance-building phase is to increase aerobic power through long, easy running. "The volume builds gradually but steadily during this phase," says Davies. Runners start with approximately 6 hours of running in the first week, with the longest run being 75 minutes. After an eight-week buildup, they have increased their weekly total by several hours, with the longest run increasing to 120 minutes. Davies prefers to prescribe endurance workouts in minutes rather than miles, allowing runners of differing abilities to follow the same schedule. He recommends running at an easy pace, or 65 to 75 percent of maximum heart rate. "Easy" for a world-class athlete might be a 6:00 mile pace, allowing that athlete to cover 60 miles in the 6 hours. Someone with less speed might run half that distance.

"The important goal of this phase," instructs Davies, "is to achieve two runs each week that last for at least 90 minutes. Wonderful changes occur to your physiology when you run for this length of time on a regular basis."

Some top athletes run twice daily to increase their weekly mileage to 100 or more. Davies endorses such an increase for the most gifted, but he doesn't recommend it for most runners. He also adds, "The

Endurance Phase

WEEK	MON.	TUES.	WED.	THURS.	FRI.	SAT.	SUN.
1	45 min. easy	50 min. easy	75 min. easy	45 min. easy	35 min. easy	50 min. easy	60 min. easy
2	50 min. easy	50 min easy	75 min. easy	50 min. easy	35 min. easy	60 min. easy	80 min. easy
3	50 min. easy	60 min. easy	90 min. easy	60 min. easy	35 min. easy	60 min. easy	90 min. easy
4	50 min. easy	70 min. easy	90 min. easy	60 min. easy	35 min. easy	70 min. easy	100 min. easy
5	60 min. easy	70 min. easy	90 min. easy	60 min. easy	35 min. easy	70 min. easy	120 min. easy
6	60 min. easy	70 min. easy	100 min. easy	70 min. easy	35 min. easy	70 min. easy	100 min. easy
7	60 min. easy	75 min. easy	100 min. easy	60 min. easy	35 min. easy	70 min. easy	120 min. easy
8	60 min. easy	70 min. easy	90 min. easy	70 min. easy	35 min. easy	60 min. easy	120 min. easy

runs prescribed here should not be shortened to allow you to handle a second run on any day." If runners want to take more time in the endurance phase than the eight weeks suggested, they can recycle through the last several weeks of the schedule. Particularly for middle-distance runners, Davies does not recommend pushing to higher mileages.

Phase 2: Hills

In this second phase of training, Davies asks his runners to include hill repeats in their training over a circuit that includes both uphills and downhills. Again, he is following the lead of his mentor. "Arthur did not invent hill training," says Davies, "but he certainly popularized this important training technique." Uphills punish the quadriceps, gluteus, and hamstring muscles while building strength. Downhills allow the runner to stretch out and build speed and flexibility. "The objective now is to build upon the aerobic phase and prepare the athlete for track workouts to come," says Davies. "Good form is important when running uphill or down. It should be likened to doing speed drills. In the endurance phase featuring long, easy running, there was no extension of the running muscles. Hill running addresses this and builds specific strength into these muscles."

Davies also believes that hill training helps balance muscle strength within each leg. "This protects runners from later injuries caused by muscle imbalances," he suggests. Although running uphill is not easy, there is less impact than when running full speed on the flat. Running downhill, of course, increases impact forces, so care must be used to run with good form during this part of the hill circuit training.

"Start by running the uphill with an exaggerated bound, driving off your toes and raising your knees," Davies instructs. "Your arms must work vigorously. Jog slowly to the gentle downhill. Run the downhill in what might be considered the classic middle-distance style: Run tall, with long strides and very relaxed arms. Your trunk should be perpendicular to the ground. You don't want to be leaning either too far forward or too far back. Run at a speed that allows you to control your movements. Don't race downhill. Jog slowly as a recovery to the steep uphill and repeat."

The ideal hill for Davies is one that is steep for about 50 meters and, if possible, adjacent to an easy downhill stretch of double that distance. "This allows you to run downhill with less pounding on your legs," he says. "You do not want to run downhill putting on the brakes." Ideally, the uphill and downhill should be approximately 200 meters apart, offering the athlete a circuit that involves running hard up and down the hill and easy at the top and bottom of the hill.

In cases where the runner cannot find an uphill/downhill combination as described, Davies suggests jogging slowly back down the uphill stretch, then doing an easy stride of about 100 meters on the flat before jogging back to start the uphill again. (In the training schedule below, a workout described as "6 × hills" would include six repeats of the uphill/downhill circuit.)

Hill Phase

WEEK	MON.	TUES.	WED.	THURS.	FRI.	SAT.	SUN.
9	6 x hills	60 min. easy	6 x hills	75 min. easy	35 min. easy	8 x hills	90 min. easy
10	8 x hills	60 min. easy	8 x hills	75 min. easy	40 min. easy	10 x hills	100 min. easy
11	8 x hills	60 min. easy	8 x hills	75 min. easy	45 min. easy	10 x hills	120 min. easy
12	10 x hills	60 min. easy	8 x hills	75 min. easy	45 min. easy	10 x hills	100 min. easy

Phase 3: Track

One of the goals of both the endurance and hill running used in the first two phases is to prepare the runner to move to the track, the arena in which he eventually will compete. Now the objective is to develop anaerobic tolerance, an ability to resist the buildup of lactic acid in the blood that inevitably forces track athletes to slow their pace. Having a high anaerobic tolerance (sometimes referred to as lactate threshold) permits you to run at a steady state for longer periods of time. In middle-distance running it is not always the fastest runners who win but rather those who can maintain their maximum speed for the longest period of time without slowing down.

Runners who reach this phase in their training will already have developed some lactate tolerance during the hill-running sessions. Track training continues the process. "Understand that this is not speed training," explains Davies. "It is anaerobic training." He advises that runners keep their speed under control. "Doing these sessions too fast can cause the athlete to reduce anaerobic tolerance rather than build it," warns Davies. (In other words, if you overtrain, you may inhibit your conditioning and/or become injured.) For this reason, he considers this the most dangerous phase of middle-distance training.

In going to the track, the warmup and cooldown now become very important. "You can't run fast unless your muscles have been properly warmed and stretched," says Davies. "Too-tight muscles increase the risk of injury." As a warmup, he recommends 10 to 15 minutes of jogging, followed by stretching and speed drills. (Speed drills consist of various types of bounding and skipping.) "If you do not know about speed drills, get help from a sprint coach," suggests Davies. "They are important for conditioning the running muscles for speed and coordination."

After the drills, he has his runners do several strides over 80 meters in the "crisp" workout zone, between 80 and 85 percent of maximum heart rate. If the wind is blowing, he has his athletes "cheat" by running with the wind at their backs to give them the feeling of running fast with less effort. After resting for 5 minutes or so to allow their heart rates to return to near normal, they begin the interval workout. After it is completed, they cool down by jogging for 10 minutes.

"Anaerobic tolerance can be developed with a variety of workouts," says Davies. "There is nothing magical about running 200- or 400- or 800-meter repetitions. If you're training for longer distances, you or your coach probably will choose the longer repetitions, but it's most important that the workout session is one that you can handle without excessive stress. Your goal is to build upon your previous training as a prelude to the final tuning phase, not to impress your coach or fellow athletes with your ability to punish yourself. That is why this phase of training needs to be individualized, with athlete and coach working together to determine what sessions the athlete reacts to best." Davies believes that this is the part of the training in which the coach can be most useful to the athlete. Self-coached athletes must take care to structure their workouts so as not to overtrain.

Other than Friday sessions in the schedule below, all sessions are done as continuous runs in which the athlete alternates fast repetitions with an interval of jogging at a slower pace. (This is where interval training gets its name.) Where the sessions are repeats up to 800 meters, jog the same distance between repetitions. (Thus, if you are running 8 × 200, you jog 200 after each fast 200.) Where the repetition is over 800, jog 800 for recovery. (In a 4 × 1000 workout, for example, you still jog 800 between repetitions.) With the faster repetitions on Friday, walk during the recovery phase.

At this point in their training, many runners feel that they need to test themselves by racing. Davies often will permit them to do so, but he warns that racing during this phase can produce slow times because of the difficulty of the training. Racing too often during any of the first three phases also can compromise the program because of the necessity to rest before and recover after the races.

Track Phase

WEEK	MON.	TUES.	WED.	THURS.	FRI.	SAT.	SUN.
13	8 x 200 medium	60 min. easy	4 x 600 medium	60 min. easy	4 x 200 crisp	1 x 2 mi. medium	90 min. easy
14	12 x 200 medium	60 min. easy	4 x 1000 medium	60 min. easy	4 x 200 crisp	1 x 3 mi. medium	100 min. easy
15	20 x 200 medium	60 min. easy	4 x 600 crisp	60 min. easy	6 x 200 crisp	3 x 1 mi. medium	100 min. easy
16	20 x 200 medium	60 min. easy	3 x 600 crisp	45 min. easy	5 x 150 crisp	2 x 1000 crisp	90 min. easy

Davies concedes, however, that high school and college runners may need to race toward the end of this buildup phase. "If so," he says, "workouts between races should be lighter." He notes that individuals differ in their abilities to handle the demands of racing programs.

Phase 4: Fine-Tuning

In this final phase, the emphasis shifts to the quality of the workouts, not the quantity. "If you want to run fast, you must be fresh, so the volume of the work is cut right down," Davies says. He notes that some athletes become obsessed with keeping their mileage high to the point that they increase the distance run during their track sessions by warming up and cooling down over increasingly longer distances. "Don't fall into this trap," he warns. "It will only make you tired and therefore slow."

Where repetitions are prescribed, walk the same distance between, unless a timed rest is given.

Fine-Tuning Phase							
WEEK	MON.	TUES.	WED.	THURS.	FRI.	SAT.	SUN.
17	8 x 200 crisp	60 min. easy	8 x 150 hard	45 min. easy	3 x 200 hard	2 x 600 hard Rest 7 min. between	75 min. easy
18	6 x 300 crisp	45 min. easy	3 x 200 sprint Rest 5 min. between	35 min. easy	3 x 120 hard	RACE OR TIME TRIAL	60 min. easy
19	4 x 300 crisp	45 min. easy	1 x 400 sprint	40 min. easy	3 x 120 hard	1 x 600 sprint	75 min. easy
20	8 x 100 crisp	35 min. easy	3 x 120 sprint	30 min. easy	Rest or 20 min. jog	MAJOR RACE	45 min. easy

Some athletes, Davies notes, take longer to develop racing form than others. "Repeating weeks 17 and 18 so that the major race is at the end of week 22 will work well. The race in week 18 could thus be an underdistance time trial over, say, 600 or 1000 meters." If runners do a time trial in practice, Davies suggests that they recruit another runner to help with the pacing.

"One important thing to remember if you are a coach," says Davies, "is that athletes are not machines. Some runners reach peak racing form quicker than others and can hold it longer. You need to individualize programs for differently talented runners. For all that we know about how to develop their physiology, we must remember that they also need to develop confidence from their training. From these schedules, you can see that the athletes are allowed to develop strength and then speed in a logical way. When they get to the final phase, they will be running fewer repetitions, which will allow them to run at a much faster pace. This is good for confidence."

Once the season ends, Davies likes his athletes to take a break from running and shift to other activities, such as swimming or biking. They then start running cross-country to prepare for the next phased training period. "Experience shows," says Davies, "that this type of formula for training will bring improved results for a three- to five-year period."

16

KIDS
COACH R'S
CHILDREN'S PROGRAM

When Marilyn Witko Rosinski trains members of the Y Junior Joggers Fun Running Club in Perrysburg, Ohio, she has them run for time, not distance. She only tells them how far they've run after they ask. Usually, the children seem surprised. "Did we really run that far, Coach R?" they ask.

"In training young children, I don't like the notion of specific distances," she says. "It's scary. They get spooked. They don't realize their capacity. Later, when they realize how far they've run, it gives them pride in their accomplishment."

When Rosinski began coaching young, age-group runners, she found that many of the children had a hard time pronouncing her last name. So she became Coach R. She had competed as a roller skater, but she married young and had four children. For several years sports were not a big part of her life. "I was living the suburban life," she recalls. "When I heard about a 10-K race in town, I thought I'd give it a try."

She eventually went on to run three marathons (her best time was a 4:06:20 in Chicago in 1991), but she devoted just as much energy to promoting exercise among her children. "My oldest son, Larry, decided he wanted to run in a CYO cross-country league," Rosinski recalls. "After his first year, the coach quit. The new coach was more interested in football, so I got involved as an assistant. Before I realized it, I was in charge of a program with 100 children, grades one through eight." (To teach others how to organize children's running programs, Coach R wrote a booklet, "Those KIDS Are Running ALL Over the Neighborhood!" Copies are available for $8, including postage, from: M. W. Rosinski, Junior Joggers, 104 Silver Maple Drive, Perrysburg, OH 43551.)

With her own children now grown, Rosinski no longer directs that program. Instead, she focuses her attention on her own Junior Joggers. "We have about 20 members," she says, "and I don't want many more than that." Because members of the club vary in age and ability, she tries to offer individual attention as much as possible. She has her young runners run "paper clips," in which the leaders loop around to rejoin the trailing group. She organizes "stagger drills," with everyone starting at different times according to ability. She talks about running like a snowball, which means starting slow and then getting faster and faster like a snowball going downhill. "That helps them stay out of oxygen debt," she says. She organizes interval workouts in which the "winner" is the runner who can come closest to running each of the repeats in the same time as his first one, regardless of how fast or slow it was. She also teaches them how to do slow-motion running, in which the object is to see how slowly they can run. "We laugh a lot," Coach R adds.

She loves it when a child comes up to her after practice and says, "Coach R, I tried what you told me, and it works!"

The Junior Joggers begin in March and continue through December before taking a break. They train hardest in summer and early fall, when the team participates in area races. She recalls running a 5-K race with a seven-year-old girl named Katie who tripped midrace and cut her hand. Coach R says, "She didn't want to quit, but she ran the rest of the race holding her hand out in front of her so she wouldn't get blood on her clean, white race T-shirt."

On another occasion Rosinski was running with a young girl who cried all during the race. "People along the route kept asking why I was forcing her to run," Coach R recalls, "but actually she was only crying because she had lost her uncle in the crowded field." That girl later went on to set state records in high school.

In teaching children, Rosinski follows a plan similar to that used successfully with adults. It's how she began when she focused on her first 10-K. It's the time-honored system of starting slow and short and gradually moving to faster and farther. Most of Coach R's workouts last 1 hour. She divides the time into three sections. The same program that she uses to train her Junior Joggers can be used by parents who are interested in teaching their children to run.

Starting Steps

Rosinski believes that it's best to establish a routine time of the day for the workout, whether in the morning, after school, or after dinner. "Whatever time works best for the family's schedule is the best time to run," she says.

She begins with a stretching routine. "This is a good time to talk and laugh," Coach R says. Her runners stretch for 15 minutes.

The second part of the hour lasts 20 to 30 minutes and combines walking and jogging. The children walk, then jog, then walk some more until they're ready to run again. Usually, beginners run several dozen steps at a time, counting out loud as they go. Eventually, they learn to run farther and rest less. She's discovered that children who have been involved in soccer programs usually are better prepared for running as a sport than children who have had no prior involvement in sports.

The third section involves what might be compared to speedwork. Coach R believes that all children can sprint for short bursts. She sets obstacle courses that involve zigzagging around trees or benches in the park. The workout's final event is a slow-motion jog to the water fountain. She finds that children laugh when they hear her say, "Slower. Run slower." Keeping track of 20 children of varying abilities is no easy task, but Coach R has been doing it for 15 years.

"The first two weeks are the 'addiction' weeks, trying to make running an enjoyable habit for youngsters," she says. "The emphasis in the run/walk segment is on increasing the length of running and decreasing the frequency of walking. Set a goal for how many times the child walks and check afterward to see if that goal is met. Walks should be long enough to avoid the stop/start pattern that wastes energy."

The following schedule should be considered as only an example of how to combine running and walking with increasing degrees of difficulty as the child begins to get in shape. On the first Monday, for instance, the child jogs or runs for 2 minutes, then walks for 1 minute before jogging again. Tuesday's workout includes 3-minute runs followed by 1-minute walks. Then the program goes back to a two-to-

The "Addiction" Weeks

WEEK	MON.	TUES.	WED.	THURS.	FRI.	SAT.	SUN.
1	15 min. stretch; 30 min. run/walk (run 2, walk 1); 15 min. fun drills	15 min. stretch; 30 min. run/walk (run 3, walk 1); 15 min. fun drills	15 min. stretch; 30 min. run/walk (run 2, walk 1); 15 min. fun drills	15 min. stretch; 30 min. run/walk (run 4, walk 1); 15 min. fun drills	15 min. stretch; 30 min. run/walk (run 1, walk 1); 15 min. fun drills	15 min. stretch; 30 min. run/walk or steady jog; 15 min. fun drills	15 min. stretch; 30 min. run/walk or steady jog; 15 min. fun drills
2	15 min. stretch; 35 min. run/walk (run 2, walk 30 sec.); 15 min. fun drills	15 min. stretch; 30 min. run/walk (run 3, walk 30 sec.); 15 min. fun drills	15 min. stretch; 30 min. run/walk (run 2, walk 30 sec.); 15 min. fun drills	15 min. stretch; 35 min. run/walk (run 4, walk 30 sec.); 15 min. fun drills	15 min. stretch; 35 min. run/walk (run 2, walk 30 sec.); 15 min. fun drills	15 min. stretch; 15 min. run/walk or steady jog; 15 min. fun drills	15 min. stretch; 15 min. run/walk or steady jog; 15 min. fun drills

one ratio on Wednesday and continues to progress through the week. A coach running along with the children quickly senses when it is time to run or walk, and the children eventually pick up the pattern.

Coaching your own child one-on-one can sometimes be difficult, particularly if the child's goals differ from yours. Coach R recommends that you run along with your child, setting an even pace and talking casually to divert attention from any initial discomfort. She says that regardless of the pattern selected, you should treat each child as someone who has individual strengths and weaknesses.

The Buildup

As the program continues, children begin to get in shape and find that they can walk less and run more during the central part of the workout. At this point in her program, Coach R begins to introduce goal-setting, both for upcoming races on the schedule and for each individual workout.

While talk about anything in general continues during the stretching portion of the workout, Coach R finds that the jogging portion is the best time to talk about running concepts. She wants her young athletes to be aware of what their bodies are doing and to understand that some generalized pain is part of the training concept. And she introduces the concept of percentage of effort: being able to run at 50 or 100 percent of your capacity at different points in a run.

As the runners become more familiar with the training routine, she allows them to help her by selecting some of the activities they want to do. They set their own target goals for the number of sprints to run during the final part of the workout. "This prepares them for goal-setting in a race," she says.

While she schedules daily workouts during the first phase, once the children become familiar with the program, they train less with the team and more on their own. This becomes their "homework." The length of runs increases from 20 to 25 to 30 and eventually 35 minutes, but rarely longer. "Exploring" involves jogging and running in new and different places.

The Buildup

Week	Mon.	Tues.	Wed.	Thurs.	Fri.	Sat.	Sun.
3	15 min. stretch; 30 min. run/walk; 15 min. fun drills	Other sports	15 min. stretch; 30 min. run/walk; 15 min. fun drills	15 min. stretch; 30 min. run/walk; 15 min. fun drills	Other sports	15 min. stretch; 15 min. run/walk or steady jog	Explore: 20 min. jog or run
4	15 min. stretch; 30 min. run/walk; 15 min. fun drills	15 min. stretch; 35 min. run/walk; 15 min. fun drills	Other sports	15 min. stretch; 30 min. run/walk; 15 min. fun drills	Other sports	15 min. stretch; 20 min. run/walk or steady jog	Explore: 25 min. jog or run
5	15 min. stretch; 30 min. run/walk; 15 min. fun drills	Other sports	15 min. stretch; 30 min. run/walk; 15 min. fun drills	15 min. stretch; 30 min. run/walk; 15 min. fun drills	Other sports	15 min. stretch; 25 min. run/walk or steady jog	Explore: 30 min. jog or run
6	15 min. stretch; 30 min. run/walk; 15 min. fun drills	Other sports	15 min. stretch; 30 min. run/walk; 15 min. fun drills	15 min. stretch; 30 min. run/walk; 15 min. fun drills	Other sports	15 min. stretch; 30 min. run/walk or steady jog	Explore: 35 min. jog or run

During winter months this second buildup phase can continue almost indefinitely. In spring or summer, with races on the calendar, it usually lasts a month.

Race Preparation

In preparing for the goal race, Coach R places the emphasis on having fun, feeling that children use their oxygen more efficiently when they run relaxed. She feels that creating runners who will continue in the sport during their lifetimes is more important than breaking records or accumulating team trophies.

By now, the children in Coach R's program have gotten in shape and become used to jogging or running for longer periods of time. Sometimes she'll surprise them by having them run a distance close to what they plan to run in the next race. She uses these surprise runs as confidence-builders, which is the reason for the use of those terms in the training table below. Workouts such as those on Mondays, which began six weeks earlier with the children running and walking, now

Race Preparation

WEEK	MON.	TUES.	WED.	THURS.	FRI.	SAT.	SUN.
7	15 min. stretch; 30 min. run/jog; 15 min. fun drills	Other sports	Surprise: 3–4 mi. easy	15 min. stretch; 30 min. run/jog; 15 min. fun drills	Other sports	15 min. stretch; 35 min. run/walk or steady jog	Explore: 35 min. jog or run
8	15 min. stretch; 30 min. run/jog; 15 min. fun drills	Other sports	15 min. stretch; 30 min. run/jog 15 min. fun drills	Surprise: 3–4 mi. easy	Other sports	15 min. stretch; 35 min. run/walk or steady jog	Explore: 35 min. jog or run
9	15 min. stretch; 30 min. run/jog; 15 min. fun drills	Other sports	Surprise: 3–4 mi. easy	15 min. stretch; 30 min. run/jog; 15 min. fun drills	Other sports	15 min. stretch; 35 min. run/walk or steady jog	Explore: 35 min. jog or run
10	15 min. stretch; 35 min. run/jog; 15 min. fun drills	15 min. stretch; 40 min. run; 15 min. fun drills	Confidence: 35 min. jog	400-meter repeats easy	Walk; talk about the race	5-K RACE	Explore: 35 min. walk or jog

blend running and jogging. Although she normally focuses on time rather than distance, Coach R will point out after certain workouts how much distance her runners have covered and compare this to the distance they'll be running in a certain race. During this phase, she discusses the race, where to pin numbers, where to stand on the starting line, and what to do when the gun goes off. Members of the Junior Joggers practice taking water and discuss what to eat on race morning.

After the race, Coach R asks the runners to describe how they felt at various points during their run. She recommends that they take any ribbons or T-shirts that they "won" to school so others can share in their excitement over a job well done.

Coach R offers the following tips for parents who are coaching their own children.

1. Keep running fun.

2. Races offer good goals, but be sure to select age-appropriate events.

3. Setting goals is important, even small goals during practice. These help put race goals into perspective.

4. Make certain that children focus on themselves as individuals, relating their success to their own abilities. Avoid comparisons with other children who may be older or faster.

5. If the training involves more than one youngster, it's important that they support each other like real teammates. This is particularly true with siblings.

6. Humor works wonders. Jokes take away the intensity of the program.

7. If you can run with your children, talking both about running and other subjects, they will appreciate the support. It shows that you feel that they are important and worth taking time for.

8. Avoid pressuring your children to meet your goals rather than theirs. Remember the first tip: Keep running fun.

WOMEN
DIANE PALMASON'S WOMEN'S PROGRAM

Do women need to modify their training programs? Do they need to be following slightly different schedules than male runners? That women do run slower than men is evidenced by the difference in the world records for 100 meters (9.84 versus 10.49) and the marathon (2:06:50 versus 2:21:06). That suggests that distances and times run in practice should also be different. But there may be other reasons that women may need to alter their training programs, including the menstrual cycle and its effects on women's moods and energy levels.

Diane Palmason raises those issues at the women's running camps that she directs with Maureen Custy-Roben each summer in Colorado and British Columbia (for more information, contact Women's Running Camp, 4029 South Roslyn Street, Denver, CO 80239; 303-

220-1037). She discovered that there were considerable differences in the ways that women felt they had to modify training to accommodate their menstrual cycles. "What surprised me," Palmason says, "is that a woman can experience quite a range of effects from her cycle. Some months, she will hardly be affected. Other months, she will experience considerable discomfort and will end up altering her training plans, either cutting back on the intensity of her workout or taking a day or two off altogether."

During Palmason's own running career, she experienced changes in her menstrual cycle, but mostly in the length and timing of the cycles rather than in any symptoms. And these variations seemed to be tied to varying levels of mileage. "Competitive stress also appeared to be a factor," she says.

Palmason, who was born in Ontario near Niagara Falls, competed for Canada in the 220-yard dash in the 1954 British Empire and Commonwealth Games in Vancouver, British Columbia. (That was the longest track distance open to women in that era.) Her best time for the 220 was 24.9 seconds.

Twenty years later, after having four children and undergoing a spinal fusion, she became aware that women finally were beginning to compete in longer distances. She was living in Ottawa at the time and ran her first road race, the National Capital Marathon, there. In 1984 she ran the marathon in 2:46:21, which was both her best time and the Canadian 45-to-49 age-group record. She holds many other Canadian age-group records at distances from 200 meters to 80 kilometers, and in 1995 she won the women's 55-to-59 age group 800- and 1500-meter races at the World Veterans Championships in Buffalo, New York.

She also works full-time coaching adult runners in person, by fax, and by e-mail. In 1990 she and Custy-Roben began a series of training camps for women runners in response to their perception that the women they were coaching had different needs and interests than men and sometimes preferred discussing those women's issues with each other.

One difference, Palmason learned during group discussions, was that women felt that their training activities were more likely to be affected in the two or three days before the start of their periods than during the days when they were actually menstruating. "The problem is both physiological and psychological," Palmason explains. "Physically, they feel bloated and heavy, since their bodies may be retaining water. Psychologically, they may feel depressed and irritable. These are typical premenstrual symptoms."

The women found that if they ran on the day their periods began, they actually felt better. "Not a hard workout, though," Palmason says, "but rather an easy recovery run."

Palmason also learned that some women's blood levels of iron seem to drop just before their periods start. Custy-Roben, confirmed this with blood tests. "She now takes extra iron. This may mean an extra serving of red meat or, for those women who don't eat red meat or are vegetarians like me, an iron supplement." (Palmason's supplement also provides vitamin C, vitamin B_6, folic acid, and vitamin B_{12}.)

"Women are more likely than men to restrict calories," Palmason says, "and in doing so, they get too little protein. Their iron needs are greater, even those who are postmenopausal. Young women also need to watch their calcium intake so that they can build maximum bone density before estrogen levels start to decrease. Postmenopausal women need even more, plus a strength-training program that stresses all the bones in the body, not just those in the hips, legs, and feet."

Palmason notes that hormone replacement therapy remains controversial, and sometimes even scary. "I've read a great deal on both sides of the rationale for taking various forms of estrogen. For those younger women who are prematurely postmenopausal because of a hysterectomy or oophorectomy (surgical removal of the ovaries), it seems necessary. I recommend that they seek the advice of a clinician who will take their running and overall lifestyle into consideration."

Most of the women runners surveyed by Palmason and Custy-Roben agreed that if they experience cramps after their periods begin, an easy run is the workout of choice. After the first day, some reported an increased level of energy and a desire to run a longer or harder workout. "The only problems then," Palmason says, "are those related to protection and comfort." Palmason advises that women wear dark shorts so that spotting won't show. Her campers felt that manufacturers of women's shorts probably need to offer a larger-than-usual "key pocket" for carrying a spare tampon. Palmason notes that Uta Pippig won the 1996 Boston Marathon while experiencing menstrual cramps, with her problem quite visible on national TV. "It didn't slow her down," Palmason comments.

The discussion with the women campers caused Palmason to reconsider training schedules, both those she uses herself and those designed for other women runners she coaches. Coincidentally, Palmason had been using four-week training cycles in her approach: A volume increase for week 1, leveling for week 2, increasing for week 3, and finally dropping for week 4, either for recovery or to taper for a race at the end of the cycle. She began to realize that this same cyclical approach could be used to accommodate the natural swings of mood and energy that women experience each month.

"The main focus and change is in the three or four days leading to menstruation and the first two days of the period," she explains. "Of course, that might mean getting away from the typical approach that the training week begins on Monday and ends on Sunday. And you would need to determine when—and if—you want to compete." There are two training programs offered here for women: One is for women who are interested only in fitness, and the other is for women who are interested in competition.

Fitness

Even though your training goal is fitness, that doesn't mean you can't train like a competitive athlete. Palmason thus recommends that women include various forms of nonrunning activities in their workout weeks. These activities include some cross-training exercises aimed at building strength, some for building endurance, and others as a form of play, what might be described as building the spirit.

Fitness athletes under her direction run only three or four days a week, but each one of those running days is done with a purpose. Rather than sending women out to run for a certain length of time at a single pace, she likes them to run varying paces, usually running fastest in the middle with a warmup and cooldown at each end. She frequently prescribes pickups, what competitive athletes might call strides or sprints. To do a pickup, you run at a fast pace for a specific (usually short) distance. After a brief rest, you run it again. A typical Palmason pickup workout would be 5 × 100 meters. The speed of the 100 meters could vary depending on your ability and fitness level. (Following the standard pace terms used in this book, this might be anywhere from crisp to sprint.) Palmason asks her runners to do pickups at the end of their running workouts, then finish with an easy jog.

"This pattern of warmup and cooldown with fast running in the middle and pickups at the end is quite familiar to anyone who has competed on a track team," Palmason says. "It's a radical way to train for women who are interested only in fitness, but it can work for them, too. Plus, once they get used to the pattern, they discover that it can be fun."

Following is the workout pattern that Palmason prescribes for the first three weeks of the month. The fourth (menstrual) week features easier training.

Monday (strength cross-training). This consists of a variety of cross-training exercises such as rowing and strength training aimed at the core of the upper body (the area around the hips and stomach). Palmason's favorite core exercise is called the Uta, after Uta Pippig. To do it, lie face-down on the floor and raise your trunk off the ground, pushing off and supporting yourself on your forearms. Hold your body straight with good form as in a push-up, except that you support yourself on your forearms rather than on your palms. Then rotate 90 degrees to the right, supporting your body on your right forearm and raising your left arm into the air. Rotate back to the opposite position, using your left forearm for support. Finally, roll over on your back and lift your hips while still supporting your weight on your forearms.

Tuesday (running). Palmason likes to structure running workouts for her clients so that they do not run everything at the same pace. In a workout lasting 40 to 50 minutes, begin by running at a slow (jog) pace for 10 to 15 minutes. Next, do a series of range-of-motion exercises that include swinging your arms in both directions as well as swinging your legs. You are now ready for faster running. In week 1, this run can be 15 to 20 minutes at an easy pace. In week 2, run 3 × 8 minutes at a harder pace with a minute of walking or slow jogging between repeats. In week 3, run 3 × 4 minutes even faster, but with a recovery period of 5 minutes. These workouts should be followed by three 100-meter pick-ups at a faster pace, with walking or jogging between pickups. Finish with 5 minutes at jog pace and stretch at the end of the workout.

Wednesday (aerobic cross-training). In contrast to Monday's cross-training workouts that focus on strengthening exercises, Palmason suggests that Wednesday's emphasis be more on aerobic cross-training exercises such as bicycling, aquarunning, and stair climbing.

Thursday (running). Thursday's workouts vary from week to week, but the emphasis is on building strength. The first week, runners do a tempo run: Begin with 10 to 15 minutes of easy running, shift into 10 to 15 minutes of faster running at a crisp pace, and finish with 5 to 10 minutes of jogging. In week 2, Palmason suggests doing a similar tempo workout, but over a hilly course with the toughest hills in the middle. In week 3, runners do hill repeats—2-minute hard runs uphill, jogging down between repeats.

Friday (rest). Palmason suggests at least one day of rest each week to allow stressed muscles to recover. For those who are unwilling to take even a single day off, she suggests walking and/or stretching with some strength work. "But don't overdo it," she emphasizes.

Saturday (endurance run). Run long, but don't necessarily run hard. Palmason suggests that you start easy and increase to a medium pace in the middle of your workout. Weeks 1 and 3 are "long" and "longer" runs, with week 2 being a tempo run. To maintain speed, run five 100-meter pickups at the end of your workout.

Sunday (cross-training). Sunday is a day of easy cross-training, featuring a variety of exercises that might be described as play. Runners are encouraged to hike, bike, swim, or go cross-country skiing. This is a day of undisciplined exercising.

For the fourth week in the training cycle, Palmason advises cutting back on hard training during the approach of menstruation, when women tend to feel lethargic. Monday is a rest day. On Tuesday and Wednesday, run for a half-hour or more. Jog the first day, and go somewhat faster the second. On Thursday, also run for a half-hour, but end the workout with some pickups, 5 × 100 meters at a crisp pace. Friday is a day of complete rest, but run a tempo run on Saturday. You should not run the middle of this tempo run as fast as you do during the rest of the month. Sunday is reserved for whatever enjoyable exercise you want to do, similar to other Sundays of the month.

Fitness Schedule

WEEK	MON.	TUES.	WED.	THURS.	FRI.	SAT.	SUN.
1	Strength	25–35 min. easy 3 x 100 pickups	Aerobics	25–40 min. tempo	Walk or rest	60 min. medium 5 x 100 pickups	Cross-train easy
2	Strength	3 x 8 min. hard 3 x 100 pickups	Aerobics	25–40 min. hills	Walk or rest	45 min. tempo 5 x 100 pickups	Cross-train easy
3	Strength	3 x 4 min. sprint 3 x 100 pickups	Aerobics	4 x 2 min. hills	Walk or rest	75 min. medium 5 x 100 pickups	Cross-train easy
4	Rest	30 min. jog	30 min. easy	30 min. jog 5 x 100 pickups crisp	Rest	30 min. tempo	Cross-train easy

Competition

For those women who are more focused on competition than on fitness, Palmason includes extra running at the expense of cross-training. "Cross-training is fine if your main goal is good health and a well-toned body. But if you want to run fast, you need to give more attention to your running muscles," she says.

The following schedule uses a pattern in which you run a competitive race the weekend before the start of your period. (That works only if you're willing to adjust your race schedule to suit your personal needs; with important races, this isn't always possible.) In dictating workouts that involve repeats, which could be run on the road or the track, Palmason prefers to use minutes rather than meters. A 5 × 2-minute workout, for example, would be the equivalent for many runners of a 5 × 400-meters workout.

Competition Schedule

WEEK	MON.	TUES.	WED.	THURS.	FRI.	SAT.	SUN.
1	Strength	3 x 8 min. hard	Cross-train	6 x 2 min. hills	Walk or rest	60 min. easy	45 min. easy
2	Strength	4 x 45 sec. sprint	Cross-train	4 x 90 sec. sprint	Rest	50 min. tempo	45 min. easy
3	Strength	5 x 2 min. hard	3 x 2 min. hard	2 x 2 min. hard	Rest	1 x 2 min. hard	**5-K RACE**
4	Rest	Cross-train	30 min. easy	40 min. tempo	Rest	Run or walk	30 min. easy

Not every woman will want to train using the combinations of speed and strength prescribed by Palmason. She understands that but adds, "You may train entirely differently on a day-by-day basis, but you can use the weekly pattern and adapt it to your own body's needs."

Palmason concedes that as a woman gets older, she may need more recovery time. "You can revise these schedules in two ways," Palmason advises: "One, by reducing the overall volume but retaining the pattern. Or two, by following a three-week cycle with two weeks of building followed by a week of recovery. If you're racing, allow more weeks between races."

18

COLD WEATHER
BARNEY KLECKER'S WINTER
TRAINING PROGRAM

Winters can be mean in Minnesota, especially when the cold winds blow from the northwest across the plains of Canada—what Midwesterners call the Alberta Clipper. The wind-chill factor sometimes dips below −70°F.

"You learn quickly to check wind direction when you head out the door," says American 50-mile record holder Barney Klecker. (He and his wife, Janis, a 1992 Olympian, live in Minnetonka, a suburb of Minneapolis.) "You'll be floating along effortlessly, then halfway through, you turn to head home and realize you're facing a 40-mile-an-hour wind." Klecker adds ruefully: "You only make that mistake once."

Yet despite what many along the Gulf Coast consider to be the world's most loathsome climate, Minnesota runners survive, and even thrive. The state boasts two top marathons, Grandma's in June and

Twin Cities in October. Its roster of past marathon greats includes Buddy Edelen, Ron Daws, Garry Bjorklund, Dick Beardsley, Steve Hoag, and the Kleckers.

Klecker believes that running through a Minnesota winter is an advantage rather than a disadvantage, because runners are compelled to change training patterns. "Winter causes a number of changes," he explains. "First, it forces you to rest a while. Second, you need to do different workouts, so you get out of the grind of 70 to 80 miles a week. There's no way you can run fast when you're bundled up against subzero winds and running on roads covered with ice and snow. You have to slow down to survive."

Klecker recommends doing indoor workouts such as treadmill running, stationary biking, aquarunning, and strength training. Outdoor workouts can include snowshoeing, cross-country skiing, or even hiking, in addition to running at a slower pace as dictated by weather conditions. Leading up to the 1992 Olympic Marathon Trials, Janis trained in that manner through a Minnesota winter. She allowed only two weeks in California for acclimatization before the late-January trials in Houston. She won in 2:30:12, a personal record.

Barney Klecker was born in 1951 on a beef and hog farm near Ellsworth, Wisconsin, and only became involved in sports when his family moved off the farm in his junior year in high school. He ran cross-country to get in shape for wrestling but soon discovered that he liked running best. At the University of Wisconsin at Stout, he ran all distances and his best mile time was 4:14.

After graduation in 1973, he worked for two years as a food and beverage director at the Hilton Hotel in Chicago and was too busy to run. He began running again when he returned to the university to attend graduate school and coach cross-country. He had run 2:43 in his first marathon several years before, but increased mileage brought his times down. In 1978 and 1979 he won the City of Lakes Marathon in Minneapolis (the predecessor of the Twin Cities Marathon), running 2:21 and 2:19.

Klecker's breakthrough came after he started training on snowshoes during the winter of 1979, mainly to get ready for the World

Snowshoe Championships, a three-day, 83-mile race. He says, "I found that the snowshoe training increased my strength and provided a break from the pounding you get running the roads." In 1981 he and his wife ran the Boston Marathon only six weeks after their respective victories in the snowshoe championships. Their Boston times were 2:16:01 and 2:40:57. "Maybe we could have run faster without having run the snowshoe race, but it didn't seem to hurt our performances," he says. Two months later, Klecker ran a personal record of 2:15:18 at Grandma's Marathon, and in the fall he set what was then a world record of 4:51:25 at the U.S. 50-Mile Championships. Without knowing the exact number, Klecker claims to have run about 100 marathons and 30 ultramarathons.

Seasonal Workouts

With four children under the age of four, both Kleckers have cut back their running mileage. Janis is a dentist, and Barney teaches at Normandale Community College in Bloomington, Minnesota. (At one time, he manufactured snowshoes, but he abandoned that pursuit because of lack of time.) They both continue to pursue snowshoeing as an alternate sport.

"We discovered that you can run extremely hard on snowshoes, but there's no pounding. The next day, you bounce right back," he explains. Another advantage of snowshoes is that moving off the roads and into the deep woods takes the sting out of wintry winds. Snowshoeing also provides such a strenuous workout that you create more body heat and stay warmer. Cross-country skiing offers similar advantages, except that you use slightly different muscles than those used in running or snowshoeing.

Nevertheless, Klecker recommends snowshoe training only two or three days a week. "If you snowshoe every day, it can shorten your stride," he admits. "Snowshoeing works best in combination with other activities." He recommends that runners include the following exercises as part of their winter training regimen.

Outdoor running. Bundle up. For maximum warmth, use layers of clothing, with moisture-wicking fabrics on the inside and moisture-shedding fabrics on the outside. A knit hat and mittens are essential. Janis sometimes wears a scarf over her mouth for protection; Barney usually just covers his exposed skin with a lubricating protector such as petroleum jelly. Don't worry about running fast; just cover the distance at a comfortable pace. The extra weight of winter clothes slows you down but adds resistance.

Indoor running. The Kleckers have a treadmill in their home that's capable of speeds up to 12 miles per hour. They can do any type of speed workout (intervals, repeats, or fartlek) that they could do on an outdoor track. Sometimes they train on the 200-meter indoor track at the University of Minnesota. Many Twin Cities runners do winter runs around the circular corridors of the Metrodome, where the Minnesota Vikings play football.

Snowshoeing. This is the Kleckers' favorite winter training activity. For fast workouts they snowshoe on packed trails (used by skiers or snowmobilers). For endurance workouts they head into the woods and trudge through snowdrifts. Klecker estimates that snowshoe miles are anywhere from 1 to 4 minutes slower than running miles. Occasionally, they don snowshoes during the summer, although they get strange stares. "Janis was coming back after a stress fracture one year and was able to snowshoe on grass two weeks before she could have started running," Klecker says. "There was less pounding."

Cross-country skiing. Although the Kleckers don't incorporate skiing into their training routine, they recognize its appeal to other runners, who sometimes shift entirely to ski trails during the winter. Cross-country skiing actually provides a total-body workout, since it also uses the shoulders and arms. "The only problem is that you do use different muscles for skiing than you do for running," Klecker says. "If you're serious about your running, you do need to mix some running with your skiing." There are two cross-country techniques, skating and classic. Skating, which is similar to ice skating in its side-to-side movements, is the preferred technique for going fast on skis. Skiers who skate need a wide, smoothly groomed trail. Classic skiing involves more straightforward movements, either in groomed, double-set tracks or in untracked snow. Classic skiing is a better cross-training technique for runners because its movements more closely resemble running.

Aquarunning. Running or swimming in a pool offers another winter option. Runners who are used to the scenery outdoors sometimes find swimming boring, but you can vary your routine by doing a variety of water exercises and even playing water games.

Stationary bicycling. Indoor biking offers a good workout while being gentle on the legs. The Kleckers do 1- to 3-minute interval sprints on the bike and find there is no residual fatigue to limit their running workouts the following day.

Strength training. The Kleckers follow a 30-minute strength routine, moving rapidly among exercises that involve 8 to 20 repetitions with relatively light weights. They alternate between upper- and lower-body exercises. It is possible to turn weightlifting into an aerobic exercise if you combine high repetitions with light weights and short periods of rest between different routines.

Winter Fitness

Many Minnesota runners use winter as a time of relaxation to recuperate from the hard training they do at other times of the year, yet they still want to maintain fitness for a quick return in the spring. Klecker recommends the following routine for maintaining fitness when the cold winds blow.

Outdoor aerobics. Activities outdoors could include snowshoeing, cross-country skiing, running, or hiking. Focus on the time and energy you spend on whatever activity you choose, not on the number of miles. Snowshoers and hikers move more slowly than runners, and accomplished skiers move faster than runners. Klecker suggests training outdoors three days a week, with one of those days a long workout.

Indoor strength. Winter is a good time to do strength training, either at a health club or at home. You can use free weights, machines, or your own body weight. Klecker suggests doing indoor strength training at least three days a week. It can be done on days when you also have other activities scheduled. For instance, come in after 30 minutes of snowshoeing to lift weights for 30 minutes. At a health club, you can run 30 minutes on a treadmill, then move to the exercise machines, and finish with a swim.

Running (outdoors or indoors). Alternate activities work well during the winter, but you also need to do some running to maintain the muscles you use in your main sport. Klecker suggests running at least three days a week, with one of those days a relatively long run.

These three disciplines can be combined as shown in the table below. On several days of the week, two activities are combined.

Klecker suggests that the following schedule should be used as a guide for winter training, not as a strict recipe to be followed blindly. Indoor and outdoor workouts—running and other activities—can be mixed, depending on convenience and the weather. "If you look out the window and discover 10 inches of fresh snow on the ground," Klecker says, "that's a day when you probably want to reach for your snowshoes rather than your running shoes."

Winter Fitness Schedule

Day	Activity	Location	Time
Mon.	Aerobics	Outdoors	30 min.
Tues.—1	Running	Outdoors or indoors	30 min.
Tues.—2	Strength	Indoors	30 min.
Wed.—1	Aerobics	Outdoors	30 min.–1 hr.
Wed.—2	Strength	Indoors	30 min.
Thurs.—1	Running	Outdoors or indoors	30 min.
Thurs.—2	Strength	Indoors	30 min.
Fri.	Rest	—	—
Sat.	Aerobics	Outdoors	1–2 hr.
Sun.	Running	Outdoors	1 hr.

Boston Bound

The Boston Marathon serves as a great attraction for runners who are able to meet its exacting qualifying standards. To qualify, men between the ages of 18 and 35 must run 3:10 in a marathon during the year before the race; women the same age must run 3:40. For men and women over 35, there is a graduated schedule of time standards that allows them 5 minutes more for every five years. With the race scheduled for the third Monday in April (Patriot's Day, a holiday in Massachusetts), runners in cold climates find themselves challenged to maintain their training buildup under difficult weather conditions. Assuming an 18-week buildup before Boston, nearly half of that training must be done from December through February, a time when the winds blow cold and footing on snow-covered streets is treacherous. The Kleckers have proved, however, that you can still run fast at Boston while using alternate forms of winter training.

Klecker's Boston-bound training schedule begins by using a pattern similar to that offered in the winter fitness program. In other words, a lot of activities besides running can be included. From the table on pages 144–145, you can pick which aerobic exercise to do on days marked "outdoors." The schedule then shifts into full-time running as the weather improves. Klecker makes several important points related to training for the Boston Marathon.

Skill level. Because of the strict qualifying standards, first-time marathoners do not run Boston. The schedule thus assumes that you are an experienced runner who is used to running 50 to 60 miles a week. If you are a first-time marathoner who is using this schedule to train for another spring race, you'll need to modify some of the time and distance goals. The schedule is designed for expert runners.

Long workouts. Through the coldest part of the winter, long workouts on Saturday are described by time rather than by distance, since you may be training on snowshoes or skis rather than running. Once the weather warms, workouts are described by distance rather than by time. Either way, the level of effort shows a steady progression upward, similar to most successful marathon training programs.

Speedwork. Once the weather warms, Klecker includes interval training once or twice weekly. Fast repeats can be done on a track or on a measured road course. In the schedule, "wup" means warmup and "cdn" means cooldown. Jog or walk 100 meters between the 100 repeats, which should be run at sprint pace. Jog 200 meters between the 200 and 400 repeats, both of which should be run at hard pace, and jog 400 meters between the 800 repeats, which should be run at crisp pace.

Hills. Unlike many of today's big-city marathons, which are held on relatively flat courses, the Boston Marathon is run from the suburban village of Hopkinton into downtown Boston on a very hilly course. Not only that, it is a downhill course. Thus, to achieve success in Boston, you need to include hills in your training. "It's important to train to run downhill as well as uphill," Klecker warns. "If you don't, your muscles won't be ready for the pounding you get on Boston's downhill stretches, particularly in the last 5 miles." Runners who live in flat areas will need to find hills somewhere. Some possibilities include highway overpasses, parking garages, stadium steps, building stairways, and treadmills that tilt. Klecker says, "Where there's a will, there's a hill."

Wake-up call. Who says training has to be easy? Most training programs offer a steady progression, and Klecker's Boston program does the same, except he asks runners to put the hammer down in week 13. He describes this week as a wake-up call. It includes 15 miles over a hilly course on Tuesday, then a 10-K race on Saturday, followed by the longest run in the progression: 26 miles. Whew! Klecker explains that the week is designed to test the mind as well as the body. "You're five weeks away. The body, at this point can handle the workload, but are you mentally ready? Do you really want to run Boston, and run Boston well?" He notes that the following week is an easy week and adds, "Remember, you're getting ready to run Boston, not the Lilac 10-Miler." In other words, wimps not wanted.

Races. Klecker is a strong believer in using races for fine-tuning in the closing stages of marathon training. He schedules six races in the last eight weeks before the final taper. He concedes that this is asking a lot of the average runner, but those qualifying for Boston are a notch above average. "This is aggressive training," Klecker admits. "The reason to

18 Weeks to Boston

WEEK	MON.	TUES.	WED.	THURS.	FRI.	SAT.	SUN.
1	30 min. easy outdoors	3 mi. easy	30 min. easy outdoors	3 mi. easy	3 mi. easy	1.5 hr. easy outdoors	10 mi. easy
2	30 min. easy outdoors	3 mi. easy	30 min. easy outdoors	3 mi. easy	3 mi. easy	1.5 hr. easy outdoors	10 mi. easy
3	30 min. easy outdoors	4 mi. easy	30 min. easy outdoors	4 mi. easy	3 mi. easy	1 hr. easy outdoors	11 mi. easy
4	30 min. easy outdoors	4 mi. easy	45 min. easy outdoors	4 mi. easy	3 mi. easy	2 hr. easy outdoors	11 mi. easy
5	30 min. easy outdoors	5 mi. easy	45 min. easy outdoors	5 mi. easy	3 mi. easy	2 hr. easy outdoors	12 mi. easy
6	30 min. easy outdoors	5 mi. easy	45 min. easy outdoors	5 mi. easy	3 mi. easy	2.5 hr. easy outdoors	12 mi. easy
7	30 min. easy outdoors	5 mi. easy	1 hr. easy outdoors	5 mi. easy	3 mi. easy	2.5 hr. easy outdoors	13 mi. easy
8	30 min. easy outdoors	6 mi. easy	1 hr. easy outdoors	6 mi. easy	3 mi. easy	3 hr. easy outdoors	13 mi. easy
9	30 min. easy outdoors	6 mi. easy	1 hr. easy outdoors	6 mi. easy	3 mi. easy	3 hr. easy outdoors	14 mi. easy
10	3 mi. easy	3 mi. wup 4 x 400 3 mi. cdn	6 mi. hills medium	3 mi. wup 12 x 200 3 mi. cdn	3 mi. easy	**10-K RACE**	18 mi. easy

race is to test your speed, particularly the 5-K races in the final month, and to test your confidence."

The schedule begins with week 1 in mid-December and continues to the Boston Marathon in mid-April.

Although runners who live in warmer climates seem to have the advantage in preparing for spring marathons, the Kleckers have proved that you can live in a state such as Minnesota and still train successfully through the winter. Boston's weather can be fickle, with

WEEK	MON.	TUES.	WED.	THURS.	FRI.	SAT.	SUN.
11	3 mi. easy	3 mi. wup 4 x 800 3 mi. cdn	6 mi. hills medium	3 mi. wup 6 x 100 3 mi. cdn	3 mi. easy	5 mi. easy	20 mi. easy
12	3 mi. easy	3 mi. wup 4 x 200 4 x 800 3 mi. cdn	8 mi. hills medium	3 mi. wup 4 x 200 6 x 400 4 x 200 3 mi. cdn	3 mi. easy	5 mi. easy	23 mi. easy
13	3 mi. easy	15 mi. hills medium	5 mi. easy	3 mi. wu 6 x 400 3 mi. cd	3 mi. easy	10-K RACE	26 mi. jog
14	3 mi. easy	10 mi. hills medium	3 mi. wup 4 x 800 3 mi. cdn	5 mi. easy	3 mi. easy	15-K RACE	5 mi. easy
15	3 mi. easy	10 mi. hills medium	3 mi. wu 12 x 400 3 mi. cdn	5 mi. easy	3 mi. easy	24 mi. jog	Rest
16	3 mi. easy	5 mi. easy	6 mi. fartlek	5 mi. easy	3 mi. easy	5-K RACE	20 mi. easy
17	3 mi. wup 4 x 100 3 mi. cdn	4 mi. easy	3 mi. wup 4 x 100 3 mi. cdn	5 mi. easy	3 mi. easy	5-K RACE	13 mi. easy
18	3 mi. easy	5 mi. easy	6 mi. hills medium	3 mi. wup 4 x 100 3 mi. cdn	Rest	3 mi. jog	2 mi. jog
19	BOSTON MARATHON						

temperatures ranging from the 30s into the 90s, depending on which way the wind is blowing. When weather conditions turn bad, the runners who are used to training in difficult conditions usually run well.

"The runner with minimal preparation can only pray for a cool day and a tailwind," Klecker says, then adds, "The will to train must precede the will to win."

19

HOT WEATHER
AL DiMICCO'S
SUMMER TRAINING PROGRAM

Training during the summer in Alabama can be tough because of a double-deadly combination of high humidity and high temperatures. Dehydration is a problem. Heatstroke is a threat. More insidious is the feeling of overall fatigue: Your body seems drained of energy. You run, but not as fast as you might under cooler conditions.

Al DiMicco, a physical therapist for HealthSouth at Medical Center East in Birmingham, prepares runners for that city's Vulcan Marathon in November by starting their training in July. To cope with hot weather, DiMicco feels that runners need to modify their behaviors. This is true whether they are training for a marathon, planning to race a 5-K, or simply running for fitness. And it can be true in the North as well as the Deep South. "I grew up in New Jersey," DiMicco says, "and it can get pretty warm there in August."

DiMicco was born in New York City in 1947 and ran high school track in River Edge, New Jersey. His fastest time for the 880 was 2:13. "I was pretty much a scrub," he admits, "but I enjoyed sports."

After attending Miami-Dade Junior College in Florida and obtaining a degree in physical therapy at the University of Alabama at Birmingham, DiMicco played handball for recreation for several years. As his schedule got more crowded, though, he sought a sport that he could do quickly during the lunch hour. He went back to running, beginning with 2 miles a day. "One thing led to another," he says, "and the next thing I knew I was lining up at the starting line of a 10-K." He ran the 1979 Vulcan Marathon in 3:14 and eventually set a personal record of 3:03. He also ran the 1995 Boston Marathon, which he calls a memorable experience. Through the end of 1996, DiMicco had completed 28 marathons and 31 ultramarathons.

In 1983 the Birmingham Track Club asked DiMicco to help with its training class for the Vulcan Marathon; two years later, he took over leadership of the class. Most years, he has two dozen or more runners in his program. He also now guides the American Leukemia Society's Team in Training in Birmingham, preparing runners for different marathons, including Marine Corps, Disney World, and Napa Valley.

Experience has taught DiMicco that runners who are planning to maintain their training during hot weather must run cautiously, taking several factors into account.

Hydration. Not only do you need to drink fluids during your workouts, you also need to drink before and soon after. "You want to make sure your water stores are topped off before you run in the heat," DiMicco advises." I encourage runners in our group to carry water bottles, either in one hand or attached to a belt," he says. "We plan our training runs so that we go by water fountains or other places where we can obtain water."

Salt. Salt helps you retain water. You can retain an additional 1 or 2 pints of fluid by increasing salt intake, which may help you get through a long run on a hot day. This causes some runners to favor a pretzel diet, but there's a trade-off. The problem is that the body quickly adjusts its hormones to balance salt levels. Whether your salt intake is low or high, within a few days, your body will readjust to normal. Most runners who have well-balanced diets probably get enough salt at meals. If you follow a low-salt or low-calorie diet, you may want to take extra salt when temperatures rise and before the week's longest run.

Diuretics. What you drink sometimes can be as important as when you drink. DiMicco discourages runners from drinking coffee the morning of their long runs. Coffee and other beverages containing caffeine (such as soft drinks) can cause excessive fluid loss through urine, so DiMicco recommends that runners drink fewer caffeinated beverages generally during the summer. Alcohol also acts as a diuretic; the higher the alcohol percentage, the greater the diuretic effect.

Headwear. DiMicco cautions against wearing a hat, since 60 percent of the body's heat radiates out from the head. "Wearing a hat is like wearing a blanket on your head," he says. "It can trap heat." But again, there's a trade-off. The sun can raise your level of heat storage by 15 percent, claims Lawrence E. Armstrong, Ph.D., an exercise and environmental scientist at the University of Connecticut in Storrs. Sunburn also can negatively affect your body's sweating ability for several days after you burn.

Whether or not to wear a hat, then, depends on *when* you run as well as what the temperature is. If the sun is low on the horizon, you'll be cooler without a hat. When running at midday under a hot sun, you definitely may want one. Caps made with mesh fabric are more effective for allowing heat to escape than those made with more tightly knit fabrics. Topless caps that consist only of visors may be best. "Running on shady courses will keep you out of the radiant sun. If you're forced to run in the sun, wetting your tank top or T-shirt (or hat) before starting will help keep you cool," DiMicco adds.

Workout time. One way to avoid heat is to run in the early morning, starting before dawn if necessary. Another is to run in the evening after the sun has set. DiMicco prefers the former option. "It's another trade-off," he says. "Humidity is higher in the morning, but there are fewer cars on the road. You're probably safer training in the A.M. than in the P.M."

Speedwork. DiMicco either decreases or eliminates most of the speedwork from his program during warm weather. "Fast running increases body temperature," he says. "It's too hard on your body, particularly for new runners." When experienced runners do run fast, he suggests that they stick to a pace specific to their race distance, whether 5-K or the marathon.

Cross-training. Training in an air-conditioned gym, either on a treadmill or on other exercise machines, is one way to beat the summer heat. Bicyclists generate their own cooling breezes as they pedal outdoors. Swimming and various aqua-exercises are other good summer options because water can cool the body and dissipate heat.

Maintaining Fitness

If you're interested in fitness, as opposed to setting a personal record in your next 5-K race or marathon, hot weather may be a time for you to retreat from the noonday sun and seek alternate training activities. Concentrate mainly on maintaining your fitness rather than trying to improve it. In this case, it's a good idea to take a conservative approach to training, especially by modifying how hard or how long you train on excessively hot days.

DiMicco's schedule uses three days a week of running as your base exercise. On three other days, you cross-train, and on the seventh day, you rest.

"If you're building aerobic fitness, the cardiovascular system cannot distinguish the method by which you stress it, only that it must improve to accept future cardiovascular demands," DiMicco states. "The intensity and time spent exercising should equate to your running intensity and time. In other words, bike at the same stress level that you might have run that day, and for the same length of time. When you run or bike, you can move your legs very rapidly, but with some machines such as a stair-climber, turnover is much slower." DiMicco recommends that cross-trainers move from machine to machine. "Use the bike and treadmill for fast leg turnover and the other machines for slower turnover and strength development," he suggests.

With the circuit training, DiMicco suggests a routine in which you warm up with 5 to 10 minutes of aerobic activity (which could be running, cycling, swimming, or walking), then move to the weight-training area. Alternate several minutes of work with free weights or exercise machines with brief bouts of stretching and aerobics, finally ending the workout with 5 to 10 minutes of aerobics. "The best exercise for finishing such a workout is probably a swim in the pool," DiMicco says. "It will both cool you and loosen your muscles."

Fitness Training

DAY	ACTIVITY	EXERCISE	TIME
MON.	Rest	—	—
TUES.	Cross-training 1 (fast turnover)	Bicycle Treadmill Jump rope	30–60 min.
WED.	Running	2–4 mi.	20–40 min.
THURS.	Cross-training 2 (slow turnover)	Stair-climber Ski machine Swim	30–60 min.
FRI.	Running	2–4 mi.	20–40 min.
SAT.	Cross-training 3 (circuit)	Aerobics Strength training	45–75 min.
SUN.	Running	3–6 mi.	30–60 min.

The 5-K

If you're interested in performance, summer is a good time to focus on shorter distances, such as the 5-K. During any workout in hot, humid conditions, body heat will rise continuously. The more intensely you train, the more quickly it will rise, and the longer you train, the higher it will rise. Therefore, to control heat, decrease the intensity or the duration of workouts, or both. If you carefully monitor your body signals, however, you can still do high-quality workouts. Here are some guidelines to keep in mind as you train.

Long runs. The purpose of running long is to develop aerobic (cardiovascular) fitness, to burn calories and control weight, to gently exercise the running muscles, and to both refresh the mind and condition it to accept stress over a long period of time. It doesn't matter how fast you run. In fact, if you run too fast, you defeat part of the purpose of the long run. So in hot weather, slow down. Slow way down. Stop frequently to drink, or carry a water bottle. Be humble enough to walk occasionally. If you are fatigued, cut the distance you planned to run. Also, pick the coolest part of the day for your long runs. If you approach each long run with a conservative attitude, you can run safely in hot weather.

Speedwork. Since running fast causes body temperature to rise rapidly, most distance runners avoid fast training during the warm-weather months. If training is done properly, however, summer can be the best time to improve leg speed. Sprinters who run 100 and 200 meters usually like hot weather because they find it easier to warm their muscles, thus reducing the danger of muscle pulls.

The secret in summer speedwork is to keep repeat distances very short and use long periods of recovery between fast bursts. If you do your speedwork at a track, you can move into the shade or cool yourself at a drinking fountain between repeats.

A typical summer speedwork session (after an easy warmup that would include jogging and stretching) would be 3 × 300 meters with 4 to 5 minutes of rest between repeats or 6 × 150 with 1 to 2 minutes of rest. The best way to run the fast splits is to run comfortably during the first third of the distance, accelerate during the second third, and finish the final third near full speed. You should finish the workout refreshed rather than exhausted. To limit stress, run your summer speed sessions very early in the day, while it is still relatively cool.

Tempo runs. DiMicco believes that if you are training to run 5-K races, you need to teach yourself to run fast for relatively short periods of time. One way to do this is by doing tempo runs, which are workouts that begin at a gentle pace, build to race pace or faster in the middle, then end at a gentle pace. In hot weather you probably want to limit the distance you run at a fast pace to no more than 1 to 2 miles out of a run that totals 3 to 4 miles. In the training schedule below, the Saturday workouts are designed as tempo runs. As with the speedwork scheduled for Tuesday, you should not finish exhausted. If you do, you probably need to limit both the distance and pace of the fast portion of your tempo runs or substitute an easy run instead.

Cross-training. The cross-training exercises in the schedule below (1, 2, and 3) are the same as the workouts described for fitness runners in the table on page 150. For runners training for a 5-K, cross-training should be done at an easy level. Consider the fact that if you decided to run instead of cross-train, you probably would jog at a slow pace to rest between hard workouts. Thus, when you move to the gym to cross-train

Hot Weather 5-K Training

WEEK	MON.	TUES.	WED.	THURS.	FRI.	SAT.	SUN.
1	Rest	4 x 150 hard	Cross-training 1	2 mi. medium	Cross-training 2	2 mi. tempo	5 mi. jog
2	Rest	5 x 150 hard	Cross-training 3	2 mi. medium	Cross-training 1	3 mi. tempo	6 mi. jog
3	Rest	6 x 150 hard	Cross-training 2	2 mi. medium	Cross-training 3	4 mi. tempo	5 mi. jog
4	Rest	3 x 300 hard	Cross-training 1	3 mi. medium	Cross-training 2	3 mi. tempo	6 mi. jog
5	Rest	6 x 150 hard	Cross-training 3	3 mi. medium	Cross-training 1	4 mi. tempo	6 mi. jog
6	Rest	3 x 300 hard	Cross-training 2	4 mi. medium	Cross-training 3	3 mi. tempo	7 mi. jog
7	Rest	6 x 150 hard	Cross-training 1	4 mi. medium	Cross-training 2	2 mi. tempo	8 mi. jog
8	Rest	3 x 150 hard	Cross-training 3	2 mi. medium	2–4 mi. jog	Rest	**5-K RACE**

on those same days, you should also work out at an easy level. Don't exhaust yourself while cross-training or you won't be able to train as hard when you return to the road or track. You also may increase your risk of injury by failing to get adequate rest as well as increase your chance of overheating if you try to push your muscles too hard to compensate for fatigue.

The Marathon

Runners in Alabama and other Southern communities seemingly have an advantage when training for spring marathons because they can run through the winter in relatively mild weather. This advantage turns into a disadvantage when they train for fall marathons, which requires a summer mileage buildup. Even runners farther north don't always find July and August conducive to weekend long runs.

Nevertheless, DiMicco believes the weekend long run to be the key to marathon success. "My program does not specify explicit daily mileage," he says. "Instead, I emphasize the weekly long run and prescribe a range of miles to be run the rest of the week, allowing runners to adapt to both their own schedules and weather conditions."

In the 22-week marathon training program on page 154, the long run is on Sunday. One day (any day) is allocated for rest. DiMicco then prescribes a mileage range for the remaining five days of the week. On two days, marathoners run 50 percent of that mileage. On the three remaining days, they run the other 50 percent. He does not care how they divide their miles as long as their total weekly mileage falls into the prescribed range.

Regardless of your personal running goals, during the heat of the summer, the body's number one goal is self-preservation. "If you ignore that," DiMicco says, "you won't meet your goals." He emphasizes that runners should plan their running routes carefully, respect the heat and sun during the middle of the day, and keep their "radiators" in good working condition by drinking before, during, and after their running and exercise workouts. With such an approach, you can achieve success training in hot weather.

DiMicco's Marathon Program

Week	Long Run Mileage	Remainder of Week
1	6	15–20
2	7	15–20
3	9	15–20
4	9	15–20
5	11	20–25
6	11	20–25
7	9	20–25
8	13	20–25
9	15	22–27
10	11	22–27
11	16.5	22–27
12	18	22–27
13	15	25–30
14	21	22–27
15	16.5	25–30
16	21	25–30
17	15	28–33
18	21	28–33
19	13	28–33
20	18	22–27
21	13	10–14
22	MARATHON	Rest

20

WALKING
MARK FENTON'S FITNESS WALKING PROGRAM

The greatest number of walkers walk just to walk, suggests Mark Fenton, editor-at-large for *Walking* magazine. "They like being outdoors," he says. "They like getting some exercise and improving their health." At the other end of the scale are racewalkers, those hip-swinging, elbow-pumping, glory-seeking individuals who have as a goal a place on the Olympic team, or at least a medal at their local walking race.

Fenton believes, however, that an additional class of walkers exists between these two extremes. These are the individuals who seek not merely health benefits but also physical fitness. They dress like athletes, not like someone out for a stroll. They walk tall, eyes forward. They take quick steps. They push off on their toes. Whether or not they swing their hips, many bend their arms and look (somewhat) like racewalkers. They probably don't compete, but walking to them is a way of life, a discipline to be pursued with some vigor—and enjoyment.

They have been described by various reporters as aerobic walkers, striders, and power walkers. Fenton prefers to use the term *fitness walkers*. He even incorporated that label into the title of a book he wrote with fellow *Walking* editor Seth Bauer, *The 90-Day Fitness Walking Program*.

"You'll get some health benefits by going out and walking at any pace, any distance, whenever you can catch time away from your work or other duties," Fenton says. "But all the scientific research proves rather conclusively that you can attain a much higher level of conditioning and well-being if you actually train to improve your aerobic fitness. Every tenth of a liter of aerobic capacity that you can cram into your body by walking farther and faster is going to increase your health and longevity as well."

Having studied biomechanics while attending the Massachusetts Institute of Technology (MIT) in Cambridge, Fenton understands walking from a scientific viewpoint. But he began as a racewalker in high school in Brockport, New York. "I started in cross-country in the fall of 1974, but New York includes the 1-mile walk in spring track," he explains. "Eventually, I competed in the state championships and in the Empire Games and was good enough to be invited to a junior national camp. That got me hooked."

Fenton attended MIT in the early 1980s, a time when the running boom was just beginning to create a spin-off walking boom. The university's biomechanical research laboratory concentrated much of its attention on research for amputees. Fenton, however, decided to focus the research for his graduation thesis on the difference in ground impact forces between walkers and runners. "My theory was that the impact with walking should be less, even in high-speed racewalking, because of reduced lifting of the center of mass above the ground on each stride," he says. That proved to be correct. "The impact each time a walker's foot hit the ground was only 1.5 times body weight versus 3 or more times body weight for runners. That suggests that walkers should suffer fewer impact-related injuries than runners."

Racewalkers who train 60 to 90 miles a week, however, do suffer overuse injuries.

That didn't prevent Fenton from continuing his career as a race-walker. He accepted a position at the U.S. Olympic Committee Training Center in Colorado Springs doing biomechanical research and also training for the Olympic Trials. He placed 10th in the 1984 trials at 50-K and was 8th in the 1988 trials. In the next few years, he continued to improve, placing 4th at the Nationals, breaking 4:20 for 50-K, and competing on the national team between 1986 and 1991. Then Fenton injured his hamstring muscles and missed the 1992 trials. "Too little stretching," Fenton confesses. "I've learned my lesson and still racewalk for fitness." He designed shoes with Reebok for three years before joining the staff of *Walking* magazine.

A frequent lecturer at walking clinics, Fenton believes one thing that separates fitness walkers from ordinary walkers (other than walking tall and bending the arms) is cadence: taking quicker steps. "Not shorter steps, but quicker steps," he says. "It's natural for your stride to lengthen a bit as you speed up, but frequency is important, too, although it's overlooked by most walkers."

The terms used in this book to describe paces for runners probably don't work entirely for walkers. Fenton suggests five paces, or effort

Walking Paces

PACE	DESCRIPTION	BREATHING	HOW TO DO IT
Stroll	"Window shopping" walking	Normal	Enjoy your walk
Easy	Continuous, comfortable walking	Almost normal	Move faster, maintaining tall posture
Brisk	Walking with real purpose	Harder, but still conversational	Think about quicker-than-normal steps
Fast	Concentrating on speed	Noticeably out of the comfort zone	Focus on quick steps and continuous effort
Very fast	Walking as fast as possible without racewalking	Near-maximum effort	Bend your arms to add speed; walk hills if necessary

levels, for his fitness walking program, stopping just short of racewalking, the heel-toe form of walking contested in the Olympic Games. The program, he explains, does not assume that you have learned to racewalk or ever intend to do so. If you feel that you can't walk quickly enough to feel the effort level described as "very fast," another option is to cover a hilly course while walking at "fast" speed. "Walking over hills increases the amount of work you do," Fenton explains, "so it increases your exercise heart rate and the conditioning effect."

In designing a program for fitness walkers, Fenton suggests that walkers build consistency, distance, and then speed.

Consistency

"In seeking consistency," Fenton says, "it is most important that walking becomes a regular habit, not something you do on the weekends or when the weather is good. The fitness walker must make a positive commitment to exercise a certain number of days a week over a specific distance or length of time, even if some of those days show fairly modest efforts." He suggests that easier days can be used when other duties demand your time.

During the first six weeks, you have two goals.

1. **Build the habit of walking six days a week.**

2. **Become accustomed to completing a variety of workouts consisting of different intensities and durations.**

Fenton defines the key to success as doing all the recommended walks, but building them into your week so that they are convenient to do. "If you have a busy day and don't have time for the 30-minute walk as scheduled, go only 15 minutes, or take the day off. Then do the missed workout on an off-day to maintain your program." Like runners, walkers should spread their more difficult workouts throughout the week rather than do them back-to-back.

If this progression seems too difficult, you can stretch the length of time by repeating weeks at one level before moving on to the next. Or if you think you are progressing too fast, you can even drop back a week before moving on. (For example, do week 3 for two weeks in a row, then drop back and do week 2 once more before moving on to week 4.) There is no requirement that you follow the schedule's timetable exactly. Your goal in this program should be fun and fitness, not getting ready for a walking race.

Building Consistency

WEEK	MON.	TUES.	WED.	THURS.	FRI.	SAT.	SUN.
1	30 min. stroll	30 min. easy	Rest	20 min. brisk	30 min. stroll	Rest	20 min. brisk
2	30 min. stroll	30 min. easy	Rest	30 min. brisk	40 min. stroll	Rest	20 min. brisk
3	30 min. stroll	30 min. easy	30 min. stroll	30 min. brisk	30 min. easy	Rest	30 min. brisk
4	30 min. stroll	45 min. easy	30 min. easy	30 min. brisk	45 min. easy	Rest	30 min. brisk
5	30 min. stroll	45 min. easy	30 min. brisk	30 min. stroll	45 min. easy	Rest	45 min. brisk
6	30 min. stroll	45 min. easy	30 min. brisk	45 min. stroll	45 min. easy	Rest	45 min. brisk

Distance

Once you have become accustomed to a regular pattern of workouts (as opposed to merely walks), you can achieve a higher level of physical fitness not merely by increasing the distance of the workouts but also by varying the distance from day to day. "You don't always need to walk the same course or the same distance," Fenton says. "Perhaps once or twice a week, set aside time for slightly longer walks, or much longer ones on the weekends." If your goal is losing weight, the more you walk, the more calories you'll burn. Walking, like running, burns approximately 100 calories for every mile covered.

Fenton describes three goals for this phase.

1. **Be able to walk comfortably for an hour at a brisk pace.**

2. **Walk as much as 90 minutes at an easy pace.**

3. **Learn to do occasional fast walks. (They are not the priority here, but they will prepare you for the next phase.)**

The key to success is to take advantage of the longer walks to maximize enjoyment. "Take longer walks in places you've never visited before," Fenton advises. "You'll have time to cover some real ground, thereby adding fun and variety to your program." He notes that many walkers discover that their long walks eventually evolve into weekend hikes.

Going Farther

Week	Mon.	Tues.	Wed.	Thurs.	Fri.	Sat.	Sun.
7	30 min. easy	45 min. easy	30 min. brisk	45 min. stroll	45 min. easy	Rest	45 min. brisk
8	30 min. easy	55 min. easy	15 min. fast	45 min. stroll	55 min. easy	Rest	45 min. brisk
9	30 min. easy	60 min. easy	40 min. brisk	50 min. stroll	65 min. easy	Rest	50 min. brisk
10	30 min. easy	65 min. easy	20 min. fast	55 min. stroll	70 min. easy	Rest	55 min. brisk
11	40 min. easy	75 min. easy	45 min. brisk	55 min. stroll	80 min. easy	Rest	55 min. brisk
12	45 min. easy	75 min. easy	30 min. fast	60 min. stroll	90 min. easy	Rest	60 min. brisk

Speed

The final element in Fenton's fitness walking program is speed. Once you have become consistent about your training and have increased the distance you walk, you can move to a higher level of achievement by improving the quality, or intensity, of your workouts. In other words, walk faster. This will allow you to improve your cardiorespiratory fitness, whether you expect to be a competitive racewalker or not.

Fenton suggests two goals for this phase.

1. Be able to walk at least briskly (or faster) several days per week.

2. Walk 30 minutes at a very fast pace every week or so, while still maintaining your weekly long walks.

The key to success is doing your fastest (and shortest) walks on your busiest days, saving your longer walks for days when you have more time. On those fast days, begin with 5 minutes of easier walking to warm up.

Increasing Speed

WEEK	MON.	TUES.	WED.	THURS.	FRI.	SAT.	SUN.
13	45 min. easy	75 min. easy	30 min. fast	60 min. stroll	90 min. easy	Rest	60 min. brisk
14	30 min. brisk	75 min. easy	30 min. fast	45 min. easy	90 min. easy	Rest	60 min. brisk
15	40 min. brisk	75 min. easy	40 min. fast	30 min. brisk	90 min. easy	Rest	60 min. brisk
16	50 min. brisk	75 min. easy	20 min. very fast	40 min. brisk	90 min. easy	Rest	60 min. brisk
17	35 min. fast	75 min. easy	45 min. fast	50 min. brisk	90 min. easy	Rest	60 min. brisk
18	45 min. fast	75 min. easy	30 min. very fast	60 min. brisk	90 min. easy	Rest	60 min. brisk

"One way to ensure success is to build some competition into your fastest walks. Consider participating in the walking division of a local 5-K or 10-K road race," Fenton suggests. "Most running races encourage walkers to participate. You don't need to try to win. Merely being part of a racing environment with large numbers of other fitness-minded individuals will guarantee that you get a good workout." Most runners consider walkers their equals, regardless of when they cross the finish line.

21

RACEWALKING
MARTIN RUDOW'S 30-WEEK
PEAK PROGRAM

At a hospital in Kalamazoo, Michigan, Martin Rudow strides across a stage in front of nearly 100 people, demonstrating proper walking technique. Rudow, a former national racewalking coach, is author of *Advanced Race Walking* (available from Martin Rudow, c/o Technique Productions, 4831 N.E. 44th Street, Seattle, WA 98105, for $13.25, which includes postage).

The hospital is Borgess Medical Center, which sponsors The Borgess Run for the Health of It! each April. The Borgess Run is actually not just one running race but a series of events at various distances, including separate 5-K fitness and racewalks. Rudow's clinic the night before the race is to teach walkers how to become better at their craft. He considers technique critical for success in his branch of aerobic exercise.

"Improve your technique, and you improve your energy system," Rudow explains. "If you become a more efficient walker, you can go faster, go farther, and get a better workout in less time. More important, better technique is easier on the joints. You'll experience fewer injuries."

Rudow describes good technique for a racewalker as having an upright posture, relaxed shoulders, a straight back, arms bent at 90 degrees, hands loosely clenched, hips swiveling naturally, and a short, quick stride with your feet rolling from heel to toe. With such movements, Olympic medals are won. Alas, despite a walking boom in the United States, Americans rarely win them. The last American to win an Olympic racewalking medal was Larry Young in the 50-K walk at Munich in 1972. Best for the United States at Atlanta in 1996 was Michelle Rohl, who placed 14th in the 10-K walk.

"Athletes in other countries don't necessarily have that much better technique," Rudow suggests, "but they're willing to train 150 miles a week. Most Americans won't make that commitment."

Like many racewalkers, Rudow began as a runner. He grew up in Seattle and ran the 2-mile in 9:42 while attending Central Washington State College in Ellensburg. He also ran 33:10 for 10,000 meters on the track, but he had already switched to racewalking by then. "I had injured my leg running," Rudow explains, "plus I liked the enthusiasm of the Seattle racewalkers, who usually were happy to share training information and offer pointers on technique to an inquiring kid."

After graduating from Central Washington in 1965, Rudow served in Vietnam as a medic and was standing in the wrong place when a shell landed. Surgeons removed more than 100 pieces of shrapnel from his body, but he recovered rapidly and placed fourth (first alternate) in the 1968 U.S. Olympic Trials at 20 kilometers. Unfortunately, knee surgery eventually ended Rudow's competitive career. "It was a congenital problem, but if I'd known more about stretching and had better shoes, I might have avoided the surgery," he says.

Because he wanted to remain in the sport, Rudow became a race official, which is not always a beloved position in the sport of racewalking since it involves disqualifying competitors for rules violations. There are two basic rules that differentiate racewalking from running. First, the walker must maintain contact with the ground at all times, with the front heel touching down before the rear toe lifts. Second, from the time the heel hits the ground to when the leg is directly beneath the body's center, the knee of the supporting leg must remain straight. "I would disqualify competitors, and they would ask me how they could improve their technique," Rudow says. "That forced me to learn what to tell them."

Proper Form and Training

Rudow offers the following tips for achieving good racewalking technique.

Posture. Keep your ears above your shoulder joints and your hips tucked under. Walk tall, looking 10 feet down the road ahead. Avoid the tendency to lean forward at the hips when going faster or up hills.

Shoulders. Keep your shoulders relaxed. Let them move with your arms. Don't try to force or swing them.

Arms. Keep your arms relaxed, bent a bit more than 90 degrees at the elbow. Drive your hands to the back of your butt and no higher than the lower part of your breastbone in front.

Hands. Keep your hands loosely clenched, but with no flopping fingers or limp wrists. You should feel as though you are driving your hands forward and back with equal force.

Lower back. Keep your back straight. Don't walk swaybacked.

Hips and lower abdomen. Keep your lower abdominal muscles gently tightened. Don't let them sag. When everything else is in line, your hips will turn naturally. Don't force them to rotate.

Thighs. Keep them relaxed.

Stride. Think about taking short, quick strides pushing off the rear foot rather than long strides reaching out with the front foot.

Feet. Focus on the heel-to-toe roll, landing on your heel with your forefoot up in front while pushing forcefully off well-flexed toes in back.

Even the best racewalking technique won't earn you a medal,

either in the Olympic Games or in your local fitness walk, unless you combine technique with proper training. In *Advanced Race Walking*, Rudow discusses technique but also offers training schedules for walkers who are interested in challenging for a medal at the 10-K, 20-K, and 50-K Olympic distances. He believes walkers in those races need weekly training mileage of at least 60, 80, and 110 miles, respectively. Rudow adds, however, that "you can still have fun, get fit, and succeed in local races with much less mileage." He suggests five days a week and 30 weekly miles as a reasonable goal for most people.

In designing a training program for racewalkers, Rudow includes the following elements.

Interval walking. This is similar to interval running, in which a hard effort is followed by an easy effort. Whereas a runner might walk or jog between fast repetitions, a racewalker would walk (or racewalk) at a slower pace between fast racewalking repetitions.

Tempo walks. These are continuous walks done over intermediate distances at a steady pace. Their purpose is to build aerobic strength, so they're done at a "crisp" pace. "Crisp" is a relative term, whether you are walking or running. Although you might be going more slowly when walking than when running, the level of effort as described in the Universal Pace Chart on page 9 would be the same. (Tempo walks, as defined by Rudow, are not the same as tempo runs as practiced by runners, which involve running at a faster pace halfway through the workout.)

Long walks. These are to build muscular strength and should be done at an easy pace. You might compare this workout to the progressively longer runs that runners do, usually over the weekend, to prepare for marathon races.

Strolling. This pace can be used on recovery days. Rudow describes it as "slower than the pace used in long walks, but you still use good racewalking technique." Strolling might be compared in degree of effort to what runners call a jog.

Rudow believes in what he calls the classical approach to training. In this approach, he lays down a base of steady training, converts to tempo work to develop an ability to hold a target pace over a long period, and finally sharpens with speed training before and during the racing season. "I suggest that racewalkers point to one target race or a series of races," he says, "and use early-season races more as training opportunities." He advises against modifying the base program to accommodate early-season competition.

In designing his 30-week training program, he uses seven set speed workouts, two each for Tuesday and Thursday and three on Saturday. Walkers can modify the schedule to do these workouts on different days of the week, depending on their personal preferences, but the pattern should remain the same. With the exception of "stroll" in place of "jog," the pace descriptions are the same as those on the Universal Pace Chart. The description of the degree of effort at which you train is the same whether you are a walker or a runner.

Rudow's Set Workouts

DAY	TIME/ACTIVITY
SAT. (WORKOUT A)	10 min. stroll 20 min. medium 10 min. stroll
SAT. (WORKOUT B)	5 min. stroll 20 min. medium 5 min. stroll 20 min. medium 5 min. easy
SAT. (WORKOUT C)	7 min. stroll 10 min. crisp 5 min. easy 10 min. crisp 10 min. stroll
TUES. (WORKOUT D)	2 x 1 mi. crisp
TUES. (WORKOUT E)	3 x 1 mi. crisp
THURS. (WORKOUT F)	4 x 800 crisp 4 x 400 crisp
THURS. (WORKOUT G)	2 x 800 crisp 2 x 400 crisp

Base Preparation

The goal of this phase, Rudow explains, is to develop the base muscular and cardiovascular strength for target races to come. "This is the best time to do cross-training," he says. "You also should take time to make any technique alterations that need to be made based on feedback received during the previous season's races." He warns that you should not expect (or seek) fast times during this phase. "Race sharpening is not important at this time of year," he says. "As you move from week 1 to week 10, you should go a bit farther each session, but with about the same effort level."

Phase 1 Training

Week	Mon.	Tues.	Wed.	Thurs.	Fri.	Sat.	Sun.
1	30 min. stroll	Rest	45 min. easy	1 mi. crisp	3 mi. stroll	Workout A	1.5 hr. stroll
2	30 min. stroll	Rest	45 min. easy	1 mi. crisp	3 mi. stroll	Workout A	1.5 hr. stroll
3	30 min. stroll	Rest	45 min. easy	1 mi. crisp	3 mi. stroll	Workout A	1.5 hr. stroll
4	30 min. stroll	Rest	45 min. easy	1 mi. crisp	3 mi. stroll	Workout A	1.5 hr. stroll
5	30 min. stroll	Rest	45 min. easy	1 mi. crisp	3 mi. stroll	Workout A	1.5 hr. stroll
6	45 min. stroll	Rest	1 hr. easy	1 mi. crisp	3 mi. stroll	Workout A	1.5 hr. stroll
7	45 min. stroll	Rest	1 hr. easy	1 mi. crisp	3 mi. stroll	Workout A	2 hr. stroll
8	45 min. stroll	Rest	1 hr. easy	1 mi. crisp	3 mi. stroll	Workout A	2 hr. stroll
9	45 min. stroll	Rest	1 hr. easy	1 mi. crisp	3 mi. stroll	Workout A	2 hr. stroll
10	45 min. stroll	Rest	1 hr. easy	2 mi. crisp	3 mi. stroll	Workout A	2 hr. stroll

Transition

During the second phase, the goal of training is to increase speed and aerobic strength. "Times become faster, and the sessions are a little harder. You should be doing all timed sessions faster by the final week." For instance, you might do Thursday's 1-mile workout in 10 minutes in week 11. By week 19, you might be walking 2 miles at that pace, or in 20 minutes. "You should expect gradual but consistent improvement over the weeks, not major jumps from week to week," Rudow says.

Phase 2 Training

WEEK	MON.	TUES.	WED.	THURS.	FRI.	SAT.	SUN.
11	45 min. stroll	30 min. stroll	1 hr. easy	1 mi. crisp	3 mi. stroll	Workout B	2 hr. stroll
12	45 min. stroll	30 min. stroll	1 hr. easy	1 mi. crisp	3 mi. stroll	Workout B	2 hr. stroll
13	45 min. stroll	30 min. stroll	1 hr. easy	1 mi. crisp	3 mi. stroll	Workout B	2 hr. stroll
14	45 min. stroll	30 min. stroll	1 hr. easy	1 mi. crisp	3 mi. stroll	Workout B	2 hr. stroll
15	45 min. medium	30 min. stroll	1 hr. easy	1 mi. crisp	3 mi. stroll	Workout B	2 hr. stroll
16	45 min. medium	30 min. stroll	1 hr. medium	2 mi. crisp	5 mi. stroll	Workout B	2 hr. stroll
17	45 min. medium	30 min. stroll	1 hr. medium	2 mi. crisp	5 mi. stroll	Workout B	2 hr. stroll
18	45 min. medium	30 min. stroll	1 hr. medium	2 mi. crisp	5 mi. stroll	Workout B	2 hr. stroll
19	45 min. medium	30 min. stroll	1 hr. medium	2 mi. crisp	5 mi. stroll	Workout B	2 hr. stroll

Race Preparation

The final phase is to get the racewalker's body ready for racing. Rudow recommends that all crisp training during this phase be done

Phase 3 Training

Week	Mon.	Tues.	Wed.	Thurs.	Fri.	Sat.	Sun.
20	30 min. medium	Workout D	1 hr. medium	Workout F	5 mi. stroll	Workout C	1.5 hr. medium
21	30 min. medium	Workout D	1 hr. medium	Workout F	5 mi. stroll	Workout C	1.5 hr. medium
22	30 min. medium	Workout D	1 hr. medium	Workout F	5 mi. stroll	Workout C	1.5 hr. medium
23	30 min. medium	Workout D	1 hr. medium	Workout F	5 mi. stroll	Workout C	1.5 hr. medium
24	30 min. medium	Workout E	1 hr. medium	Workout G	5 mi. stroll	Workout C	1.5 hr. medium
25	30 min. medium	Workout E	1 hr. medium	Workout G	5 mi. stroll	Workout C	1.5 hr. medium
26	30 min. medium	Workout E	1 hr. medium	Workout G	5 mi. stroll	Workout C	1.5 hr. medium

just below the target pace that you expect to achieve in races. But he also warns, "Be ready to back off workout intensity if you develop any aches and pains. The base training will see you through any downtime." He expects that racewalkers will see a definite improvement in all times and distances between the first and last weeks of this phase.

The Racing Season

"During this period, the goal is mainly to maintain conditioning," Rudow says. "Even if you race every weekend, you can maintain your level if you cut your training between races." Although the following table demonstrates training over a period of four weeks, encompassing races of varying distances, racewalkers can adapt the basic pattern shown in week 27 for any number of weeks, depending upon their race schedules. Week 30 suggests a taper before an important 10-K race, one that you have chosen for your season's peak performance.

			Racing				
WEEK	**MON.**	**TUES.**	**WED.**	**THURS.**	**FRI.**	**SAT.**	**SUN.**
27	Rest	3 mi. crisp	1 hr. medium	3 x 800 hard	Rest	**5-K RACE**	30 min. stroll
28	Rest	3 mi. crisp	1 hr. medium	6 x 400 hard	Rest	**8-K RACE**	30 min. stroll
29	Rest	3 mi. crisp	1 hr. medium	3 x 800 hard	Rest	Workout B	30 min. stroll
30	Rest	3 mi. crisp	1 hr. medium	30 min. stroll	Rest	**MAJOR 10-K RACE**	Rest

Rudow believes that the 30-week program offers racewalkers a new and different approach to their sport. "If you want to achieve peak performance, it will give you great dividends," he comments.

Although the schedules in this chapter were designed for racewalkers, they also could be modified to accommodate the training of runners. This is true particularly because most of the workouts are described in minutes rather than miles. Similarly, walkers who are looking for training variations can modify many of the running programs in this book to accommodate their needs.

22

THE TRIATHLON
HANK LANGE'S TRIPLE-THREAT PROGRAM

Hank Lange insists that skiers were the first cross-trainers. "We had to be," he says. "There's no snow in summer, so we ran, biked, and lifted weights to stay in shape."

Born in Schenectady, New York, Lange competed in swimming in high school and switched to cross-country skiing while attending Bowdoin College in Brunswick, Maine. While at Bowdoin (Joan Benoit Samuelson attended at the same time), Lange was named to the NCAA Division II All-East ski team three times. After graduating in 1975 with a degree in economics, he coached cross-country skiing at Bates College in Lewiston, Maine, and later at Keene State College in Keene, New Hampshire. He also served as a coach for the U.S. Ski Team. (Among the skiers he coached at Bates was Nancy Fiddler, a 17-time national champion and two-time Olympian.) When the triathlon emerged as an important sport in the 1980s, Lange realized that his background offered an excellent springboard into an event that features swimming, bicycling, and running.

The most popular distances for the triathlon legs, and the ones recognized internationally, are a 1500-meter swim, a 40-kilometer bicycle ride, and a 10-kilometer run. Triathlon distances can be shorter or longer, however. The exclusive Ironman Triathlon in Hawaii features a 2.4-mile swim, a 112-mile bike ride, and a 26.2-mile run.

Lange, who now lives in Brattleboro, Vermont, placed 20th at the Ironman in 1982 and competed for four years on the Saucony Triathlon Team. At the 1994 World Triathlon Championships in Wellington, New Zealand, Lange won the bronze medal in the 40-to-44 age group. He has won 23 triathlons and medaled in more than 100 endurance events. A certified coach in swimming and cycling, he has coached triathletes to world and national age-group titles.

Less Is More

While many champion triathletes train up to 8 hours a day to achieve success, Lange believes that you can participate in triathlons and still have a real life. In fact, you may be able to achieve *greater* success by doing less rather than more. "While I was still experimenting with my training, I experienced some notable failures," he admits. "I'd go into an event seemingly in great shape and crash badly. After doing well at Ironman, I increased my training the following year and failed to make the start. I was overtrained. It took me a while to sort that out."

Armed with knowledge gleaned from his own mistakes, Lange makes certain that the adult athletes he now coaches through his firm, Personal Best, do not try to substitute tenacity for intelligence. "Just because you run 7 hours a week doesn't mean you add 7 hours of swimming and 7 hours of bicycling when you become a triathlete," he says. "You run out of hours fast that way. It's better to take those 7 hours and allocate time to each of the three events in combination with each other." He concedes that triathletes do need extra training time, but he believes that extra hours are best used when focused on technique rather than endurance. "Work on your weaknesses rather than your strengths," he says.

What are the necessary ingredients for success in the triathlon? Lange points to four areas (the three activities plus the transitions between them).

Swimming. Technique is more important in swimming than in any other triathlon event. Arm strength and endurance are needed, but unless you know how to pull yourself through the water efficiently, you'll quickly fall behind those with smoother strokes. "You need to learn to relax all your muscle groups," Lange says. "Being supple is better than being strong." Despite his background as a swimmer, when Lange switched to the triathlon, he went to the swim coach at Keene State College for help with positioning himself in the water. Tip: Wearing a wetsuit helps novice swimmers work on their stroke dynamics and allows them to float higher in the water.

Bicycling. Technique when riding a bike may seem less important, but it can still save you time. "It's not only aerodynamics," Lange says. "You need to be in a position to deliver power to the wheels and yet remained relaxed." He says that he sees novice riders with saddles too low or with frames too big. One way to avoid this is by seeking help at a local bike shop. Equally important is cadence, or how many revolutions a minute you spin your wheels. Spinning at too low a cadence in too high a gear wastes more energy than the proper cadence (85 to 95 revolutions per minute) in the proper gear. Lange finds that many runners bike at too low a cadence and too high a gear when moving from their regular sport to the triathlon.

Running. Being trained to run is not enough. Equally important is attaining a quick and efficient stride once the running begins. "That's not easy," Lange admits. "In a normal 10-K, you have time to warm up. In a triathlon, you're both fatigued from the swim and stiff from the bike ride before you start to run. You can waste a lot of time and energy in the first few miles unless you teach your body to switch fast into its running mode. Also, avoid overstriding."

Transition. To achieve that efficient switch, Lange recommends that triathletes practice transitions. In designing programs, he schedules several dual-sport workouts a week, where the emphasis is on moving quickly from one sport to the other. "In the swim, your body has been shunting blood flow to the shoulders and the arms. Suddenly you're biking, and the blood has to come down to the legs. You can blow your quads unless you learn to make that shift smoothly." He notes that not only is the transition physical, it is mental. "I often see triathletes wandering around the corral after the swim because they can't remember where they've parked their bikes. You need to practice the little things, like tying shoes and changing clothes. If you wear a wetsuit for warmth and buoyancy, you'd better learn how to get out of it rapidly."

The triathlon is an event in which an ability to purchase increasingly expensive equipment, like wetsuits and light bicycles, can allow triathletes to trim their times, sometimes significantly. But at the upper reaches of the sport, everybody uses the best equipment. "Inevitably," Lange says, "there's no substitute for training." He has designed a 10-week program that allows runners to shift from their regular sport to the triathlon. While designed for those interested in competition, Lange's training patterns can also be used by runners whose only desire is cross-training for a higher level of fitness, without ever going near a triathlon starting line.

The Buildup

Before beginning this buildup, you should already be proficient in your main sport of running. This means that you should be training at least 20 to 30 miles a week and be capable of participating in 5-K and 10-K races without undue stress. To prepare for the standard distance, Lange suggests that you train at least six days a week, combining two sports in a single workout on several days. If you take a day off, he recommends that you skip a day on which your strongest sport (running) is scheduled, because that's where you'll lose the least. If you miss an occasional second workout, or one devoted to recovery, the rest will often do you good. "Technique is paramount," he emphasizes. "And you can't work on technique if you're fatigued from too many hours of training." Here are the elements of the buildup phase.

Warmup and cooldown. Start the swim workouts with 5 to 10 minutes of easy swimming to warm up before the faster work. Afterward, do a similar cooldown to relax your muscles. Warmups and cooldowns work well in bicycling and running, and they can be included as part of the time allotted for the workouts.

Speed drills. Lange recommends speed drills to enhance speed and technique in each of the three triathlon disciplines. Whether stroke drills in swimming or spinning drills on a bike, these are best learned from a good coach. "Golfers, skiers, and tennis players accept the fact that they can improve their skills by taking lessons," he says, "but swimming, bicycling, and running seem so natural that many people think they won't benefit much from coaching. That's not true." Learning technique in all three sports is essential to triathlon success.

Double sports. On several days Lange combines workouts in two sports, such as 30 minutes of swimming leading into 30 minutes of bicycling. Moving fairly quickly from one sport to another allows you to practice transitions, which are essential in racing. Thus, you would train by swimming first and biking second, or biking first and running second. On days when you run or bike long, you might want to reverse the process by finishing your workout with an easy swim or by spinning on an exercise bike. That serves as a cooldown and will help relax your muscles.

Pickups. Fartlek is an important form of speed training for runners in which they run at different paces for different distances. Pickups are similar in that you bike or run at a steady pace, picking up the pace for different periods of time. In training, there are occasions when it is best to let your body and mind dictate changes in pace rather than following a set pattern. This is one such occasion.

A typical 30-minute bike ride with pickups might work like this.

- **10 minutes easy**
- **10 minutes, alternating hard and easy, with 40-second recovery periods**
- **10 minutes easy**

Strength and stretching. Lange considers strength and flexibility training essential to success. These are best done at the end of a workout when your muscles have been warmed. For stretching, Lange favors yoga, a discipline that involves static stretching. "This is particularly important because bicycle riders must learn how to remain relaxed while staying in the same position," he says.

Lange suggests a steady buildup for the first 6 weeks of his 10-week program leading to a peak triathlon. The workout pattern remains the same for this period, but the numbers change, progressing upward. On days where the prescription is for 20 to 40 minutes of exercise, begin with 20 minutes the first week and build toward 40 minutes by the sixth week.

Six-Week Buildup Phase

Day	Swim	Bike	Run	Other
Mon.	5 min. warmup 10 min. drills: 10 x 50 hard 5 min. cooldown	—	—	Strength training
Tues.	—	20–40 min. easy	20–40 min. medium	Stretching
Wed.	10 min. drills: 3 x 100 hard 2 x 200 crisp 2 x 50 sprint	—	30 min. easy w/pickups	Stretching
Thurs.	—	40–60 min. w/pickups	—	Strength training
Fri.	—	—	Rest or easy run	Stretching
Sat.	30 min. easy	1–3 hr. easy	—	Stretching
Sun.	—	Spin drills	1–2 hr. easy	Stretching

The Tuneup

The focus in the last four weeks is on increasing the level of effort. Lange, however, stresses that even on hard days, you should not push past the point where you feel tension in your muscles. Give extra emphasis on Tuesday (when you bike and run) to the transition between those two events, which is a trouble spot for most novice triathletes. He reserves the weekends for a mixture of distance running to keep up your strength and long bike rides to maintain your power and endurance. In the eighth week, run a 10-K race as a test of your general fitness.

Four-Week Tuneup Phase

Day	Swim	Bike	Run	Other
Mon.	3 x 500 easy to hard	—	—	Strength training
Tues.	—	5 x 1 mi. medium	4 mi. tempo run	Stretching
Wed.	10 min. drills 5 x 200 medium	—	40 min. easy w/pickups	Stretching
Thurs.	—	60–90 min. w/pickups	—	Strength training
Fri.	—	—	—	Stretching
Sat.	10 min. drills 2 x 1000 easy	Spin drills	90 min. easy	Stretching
Sun.	—	2 hr. easy	30 min. medium	Stretching

In the final week, taper by cutting distances but maintaining intensity. Most runners switching to the triathlon discover that finishing the standard 1500-meter/40-K/10-K is no more difficult than finishing a marathon, provided they train properly in the other two sports. Moving up to the distances used in the Ironman Triathlon, an event that takes competitors 8 or more hours to finish, demands a different approach to training and considerably more time.

23

POWER
VERN GAMBETTA'S
STRENGTH-TRAINING PROGRAM

Vern Gambetta played football at Fresno State University in California and also competed in the decathlon in track and field. "I trained with a lot of good people, including Bill Toomey (1968 Olympic champion)," Gambetta says, "but I was about 2,000 points behind him."

Yet as a coach, Gambetta has had some of his greatest success coaching long-distance runners. His girls' cross-country team at Santa Barbara High School went undefeated from 1975 through 1977. The 1977 girls' team set a national high school distance medley record. That same year, he had six boys run faster than 10 minutes for 2 miles, four of them under 9:27. Between 1977 and 1982, he served as head coach for women's track and field and cross-country at the University of California at Berkeley. His 1982 track team placed second at the national collegiate championships. He also served as first director of The Athletics Congress Coaching Education Program, which is designed to upgrade the standard of track-and-field coaching in the United States.

After leaving college coaching, Gambetta served as director of conditioning for the Chicago White Sox baseball team and also worked with the Chicago Bulls basketball team. Now living in Sarasota, Florida, Gambetta continues to train athletes as president of his own consulting firm, Gambetta Sports Training Systems. His current clients include the Tampa Bay Mutiny, a professional soccer team. He has written three books, including *The Complete Guide to Medicine Ball Training*.

Radical Move

"As a decathlete, I always approached running from the perspective of speed and power rather than endurance," Gambetta says. "I've continued that approach as a coach. Strength training is well-accepted as an adjunct to any well-rounded training program for distance runners today. When I first started having my distance runners use barbells in the 1960s, it was considered a radical move."

Gambetta, however, notices that while distance runners at the elite level embrace strength training as a necessary means for achieving peak performance, recreational athletes often pass the weight room by. "If it's the difference between a gold and silver medal at the Olympic Games, or even getting to the Olympic Games, you're going to take the extra time to train your body," he says. "Most elite runners are full-time professionals anyway. They train twice daily, 3 or 4 hours a day, sometimes under the supervision of a knowledgeable coach. If they don't have the disposition for strength training, their coaches will tell them what to do."

A busy physician or accountant who is trying to find some time to run before catching the commuter train home may find that it's simpler and easier to just run, even though adding a minimal amount of strength training might result in faster 10-K or marathon times.

"The key to good performance is posture," Gambetta says. "The best distance runners have very upright postures, efficient arm carriages, and smooth strides, neither too short nor too long. Strength training can improve posture by increasing the strength of the central body core on which your arms and legs are anchored. Strength training can also promote joint stability and prevent injury."

But can a busy executive gain enough from strength training to justify the 15 or so minutes two or three times a week that he might be willing to add (or subtract) from his running time? "I don't believe a world-class runner can succeed with 15 minutes of strength training," Gambetta says. "But even that much commitment would help a recreational runner begin to perform better by helping to improve mechanical efficiency as well as preventing common injuries."

Periodization

One secret to both increasing and maintaining strength is periodization, a buzzword that refers to using different training programs for different periods of the year and a series of progressions, or steps, in which athletes move from one level of fitness to another. While that busy executive might not want to divert time from his running to do strength training when the weather is nice, cold winds and snow may make a workout indoors pumping iron more attractive.

"If you can build your strength by putting in some 30-minute days in the weight room three or four days a week during what distance runners might call the off- or building season," Gambetta adds, "then you can maintain your strength with somewhat less work at other times of the year. If you're at the peak of your marathon training and doing 15- and 20-mile runs on the weekend, maybe you shouldn't be diverting too much more of your energy to work with the weights. It might even increase your risk of injury or the other bad effects that come with overtraining. But once that marathon is over, and while you're deciding on your next training goal, that's the time to increase your strength-training commitment, because it will help you with whatever you select as that next goal—even if that goal is only general fitness and good health."

Gambetta feels that all the multijoint movements of the legs can be trained with a few very simple exercises. He suggests two or three days a week of strength training as appropriate for runners. Strength can be achieved by various means, including exercise machines and free weights, or simply by calisthenics-type exercises as simple as pull-ups and push-ups. Gambetta is not a fan of sit-ups, because he feels the straight-up-and-down motion does less to strengthen the central body core than others he might recommend, such as training with a medicine ball. (Also low on the Gambetta scale of training effectiveness for distance runners are machine or barbell exercises in which you push the weight overhead, such as the military press.)

Gambetta tries to avoid exercises, such as the bench press, that might increase upper-body mass, thus giving the runner more weight to carry while running. He also believes that you cannot divorce strength from flexibility. "A good strength program promotes dynamic flexibility," he says. (With his professional athletes, he teaches flexibility by having them walk and sidestep with a 9-inch-long rubber band on their ankles.)

"The goal is to condition you to run in order to optimize training time," Gambetta says. "The program involves a lot of work, but if followed in a progressive manner, it will yield great results."

Flexibility and Balance

The most effective time to stretch is after each run and after each strength session to restore muscles to their resting length. "Stretching before a run or a workout without a previous warmup is very ineffective," Gambetta says. He identifies the areas that need particular attention as the quadriceps, hamstrings, shins, and calves. Another area that is often overlooked is the iliotibial band, which stretches from the hip to the knee. It acts as a major stabilizer of the knee; if flexibility of the iliotibial band is not addressed, in high-mileage situations, it can cause knee pain, which can restrict running. He recommends stretching all of these muscle groups daily to enhance performance and prevent injury.

Runners must work on balance to develop stabilizing muscles and to improve body awareness. This will help avoid common overuse injuries, such as Achilles tendinitis and plantar fasciitis. Gambetta recommends single-leg squats. To do them, balance on one leg, with that leg in a flexed (bent) position and the other leg held high. Do each of the following positions twice for each leg and hold for a count of 10.

- **Straight behind (extend the second leg behind you)**
- **Side (hold the second leg out to the side)**
- **Rotation (move the second leg from front to back and back to front)**

Gambetta suggests including this balance routine in your warmup and cooldown each day you run.

Core Work

Gambetta believes a strong core (hips, abdomen, and lower back) to be extremely important in maintaining good running posture. The following abdominal exercises should be done while lying on your back on the floor. Repeat each exercise 20 times.

Leg raises. While lying on the floor with your hands placed under your pelvis for stabilization (and to take the curve out of your lower back), bend your knees slightly and raise and lower your legs 18 to 20 inches.

Lower-abdominal sit-ups. Lying in the same position as for the previous exercise, bring your knees toward your chest and point your feet toward the ceiling.

Curl-ups. Lie with your knees bent, your feet flat on the floor, your arms folded across your chest, and your chin tucked in. Gradually lift your body between your butt and shoulders (imagine that you are doing so one vertebra at a time) until your trunk is flexed 30 degrees off the floor. Lower your body slowly.

Crunches. Lie with your knees bent, your thighs perpendicular to the floor, and your calves and feet parallel to the floor, supported by a chair or a bench. With your arms on your chest, gradually begin to curl your body up off the floor, again imagining that you are lifting one vertebra at a time, until your trunk is flexed 30 degrees off the floor. Lower your body slowly.

Twisters. In the same position as for the previous exercise, lock your hands behind your head. Curl up and twist, touching your right elbow to the outside of your left thigh. Lower your body, then curl up and touch your left elbow to the outside of your right thigh. Lower your body slowly.

Generally, Gambetta, prefers that runners stand while exercising the core, since this allows natural hip movement. It also takes better advantage of the effect of gravity. For equipment, use a medicine ball or your own body weight. "Traditional exercises in the lying position, where the pelvis is less fixed (such as sit-ups), are less functional and should occupy a smaller proportion of the training time," he comments.

The following medicine ball rotations should be done while standing with your feet shoulder-width apart, or slightly wider, and your knees slightly flexed. Use a standard medicine ball. Except where noted, each exercise should be repeated 10 times.

Tight rotations. Holding the ball directly in front of your navel and close to your body, rotate as far to the right as possible, then immediately rotate to the left. Rotate your hips as though swinging a golf club.

Wide rotations. This is similar to the previous exercise, but begin by holding your arms extended in front of you from the waist and swing the ball in a wide arc.

Waist chops. Start by holding the ball overhead and off to one side. With a chopping motion, bring the ball down and across to your hip on the opposite side.

Knee chops. This is similar to the previous exercise, but bring the ball down and across to the opposite knee.

Ankle chops. Again, a similar exercise, but this time bring the ball down and across to the opposite ankle. Stand up completely after each repetition and reach as high as possible with the ball. (Repeat 5 times instead of 10.)

Woodchopper twists. Start by holding the ball over your head. With a chopping motion, bring the ball straight down between your legs, as though you were chopping wood. Then straighten up, reaching as high as possible, and twist either right or left after each repetition.

Strength Work

Gambetta designed the following program to target upper-body muscles that enhance good running posture. The last two exercises require the use of dumbbells.

Push-ups. These should be done in both the regular push-up position (back straight) and the bent position (butt up). Do 20 repetitions each.

Pull-ups. Hold on to the bar with your hands facing away from you. Do 10 repetitions.

Rhomboids. Lie face-down on a bench and hold two dumbbells to the sides, then pull them toward your chest. Do 10 repetitions.

Dumbbell shrugs. Standing upright, hold the dumbbells at your sides and shrug your shoulders. Do 10 repetitions.

Gambetta believes in training each leg separately, in most cases using only your own body weight. "If you're a 150-pound runner, you get more resistance by lifting that body weight with one leg than with two," he says. "Also, if you lift with two legs, there's a tendency to favor one leg, shifting some of the weight onto one leg rather than the other. One-leg lifts allow you to give each leg equal attention."

Because runners use their legs regularly as they run, Gambetta does not advise strength training them as frequently as the trunk and upper extremities. He considers two days in a seven-day cycle sufficient. He suggests first using only your own body weight and the force of gravity. Later, you may want to add extra weight to increase resistance. (The squats below should actually be half-squats in which you lower your trunk only halfway to the floor.)

Single-leg squats. Do 10 repetitions each with the trailing leg first held straight to the front, then to the side.

Double-leg squats. Do 20 repetitions with both legs.

Lunges. Standing with your legs together, lunge forward with one leg. Do 10 repetitions with each leg.

Step-ups. Standing on the floor in front of a step 12 or 15 inches high, step on and off, beginning with the same leg each time. Do 10 repetitions with each leg.

Starting Out

The goals of the base program below are to establish a routine and learn how to do the exercises correctly and in combination with your running. This schedule is the type that a beginning runner might follow, or an experienced runner who has begun to integrate strength training into his normal running routine.

Each day features a different mix of the various strength exercises described earlier. Stretching is not included, but you should stretch each day. "Abs" and "back" refer to exercises described in the section on core work. The running workouts merely suggest how to pattern your running in combination with your strength training. Precisely what you run depends on which specific schedule (such as those elsewhere in the book) you're following.

Base Routine						
MON.	**TUES.**	**WED.**	**THURS.**	**FRI.**	**SAT.**	**SUN.**
Balance	Balance	Balance	Balance	Balance	Balance	—
Abs	Medicine ball	Medicine ball	Medicine ball	Medicine ball	Back	—
Legs	Upper body	Medicine ball	Legs	Upper body	Medicine ball	—
—	Run easy	—	Run easy	—	Run easy	Run easy

Building Strength, Endurance, and Power

Once the strength exercises have been integrated into your running program, the next goals are to increase the volume of exercises and shorten the recovery period between them, both in your strength training and in your running workouts. The following schedule might be used by a runner who trains for fitness, not for competition, or by an experienced runner who is beginning to increase his level of strength training.

Strength and Endurance Routine

Mon.	Tues.	Wed.	Thurs.	Fri.	Sat.	Sun.
Balance	Balance	Balance	Balance	Balance	Balance	—
Back	Back	Abs	Back	Back	Abs	—
Legs	Upper body	Medicine ball	Legs	Upper body	Medicine ball	—
—	Run easy	Run hard	Run easy	—	Run easy	Long run

The goals with the next routine are to raise power levels and train to sustain them. This schedule might be used by a runner who uses a sophisticated running schedule to prepare for competition. As above, the running workouts below are merely to suggest a pattern of training.

Power and Endurance Routine

Mon.	Tues.	Wed.	Thurs.	Fri.	Sat.	Sun.
Balance	—	Balance	—	Balance	—	—
Back	Back	Abs	Back	Back	—	—
Legs	Upper body	Medicine ball	Legs	Medicine ball	Medicine ball	—
Run easy	Tempo run	Run easy	—	Run medium	Speedwork	Long run

The following strength workouts can be used when exercising the legs or upper body in both of the schedules above.

For the legs:

- Single-leg squats: 3 × 10 reps (each leg, both positions)
- Double-leg squats: 3 × 20 reps
- Lunges: 3 × 10 reps (each leg)
- Step-ups: 3 × 10 reps (each leg)

For the upper body:

- Push-ups: 3 × 20 reps (both positions)
- Pull-downs or pull-ups: 3 × 12 reps

- **Rhomboids:** 3 × 10 reps
- **Dumbbell shrugs:** 3 × 10 reps

Racing

As you get closer to racing, the goal shifts to sharpening your skills by taking advantage of the work done so far. This is the taper phase in strength training, and the emphasis is on more explosiveness. "Everything is geared toward racing to win," Gambetta says.

Taper Routine						
MON.	**TUES.**	**WED.**	**THURS.**	**FRI.**	**SAT.**	**SUN.**
Balance	Balance	Balance	Balance	Balance	Balance	—
Back	—	Abs	Back	—	—	—
—	Legs/ upper body	Medicine ball	—	Legs/ upper body	Medicine ball	—
Tempo run	Run easy	—	Speedwork	Run easy	—	**RACE**

In this final tapering phase, Gambetta combines the strength training for the legs and upper body into a single workout to be performed two days during the week.

- **Single-leg squats:** 10 reps (each leg, both positions)
- **Lunges:** 2 × 10 reps (each leg)
- **Step-ups:** 2 × 10 reps (each leg)
- **Push-ups:** 20 reps (both positions)
- **Pull-downs or pull-ups:** 2 × 12 reps

Gambetta believes that only by including strength training in their daily routines can runners train effectively and maximize their chances for success. "By becoming stronger, you can run stronger," he says. "It's that simple."

24

COMING BACK
BOB WILLIAMS'S REHAB
PROGRAM

When one of his runners gets hurt, Bob Williams often feels the pain as much as the athlete. "It always has been my goal to coach runners to avoid injury," says the Portland, Oregon, coach. "I take pride in the fact that the runners I coach seldom are injured or sick. I educate them constantly on how to not get hurt. So when something goes wrong, I feel responsible."

Fortunately, Williams is among the most knowledgeable coaches when it comes time to rehabilitate runners after an injury. He learned his coaching trade from the master: He ran at the University of Oregon under legendary track coach Bill Bowerman and competed in the 3000-meter steeplechase, an event he ran in both the 1968 and 1972 U.S. Olympic Trials. (He placed fifth in 1968 with a time of 8:41.2.)

Currently, Williams serves as a sports medicine specialist at Portland Adventist Medical Center. A successful coach of adult runners, he also helps supervise a Portland Marathon training class that attracts more than 200 participants each year.

"Every runner is going to get injured to some degree at some point in his career," Williams says. "What you do with your rehabilitation determines how quickly you get back in shape and how successful you are at avoiding future injuries."

Some injuries (such as stress fractures) require total abstinence from running. With others, the athlete may be able to continue running but at a much-reduced level. Before permitting his athletes to return to running at full speed again, Williams insists that they be symptom-free. That means no pain in the injured area when they perform weight-bearing exercises such as running or even walking. "You can do anything as long as you're symptom-free," he says.

The worst mistake any runner can make while rehabilitating from an injury, Williams believes, is to start running again too soon or too hard. "The danger there is that not only can you reinjure yourself, but in favoring the original injury, you can create additional problems. While favoring a sore ankle, you run with an awkward stride, which causes you to injure a knee or a hip. Second injuries cause more problems than the first ones. They're often more difficult to treat."

To offer his runners a guide to help avoid reinjuring themselves, Williams has developed a pain index by which they can rate how much the injury hurts on a scale of 0 to 5. That allows them to monitor their own levels of rehabilitation and to determine whether to run or not run and whether to cross-train or avoid exercise entirely.

Rehabilitating runners often experience different levels of pain at different points during a run. By warming up carefully and not pushing too hard at the beginning of the workout, a runner with a mild injury sometimes finds that the pain will disappear, allowing him to run faster toward the end. On other occasions, he may begin the run feeling good, only to have the pain worsen as he completes the run.

"The most important factor is whether or not the pain index numbers are coming down or going up," Williams says. "If you begin the

Williams's Pain Index

DEGREE OF DISCOMFORT	DESCRIPTION	STRATEGY
0	No pain	Free to run
1	Some discomfort after run	Flat, soft surfaces only
2	Uncomfortable before run	Walk first, then jog
3	Somewhat painful	Walking only
4	Very painful	Don't even walk
5	Extremely painful	Call 911

workout with a 3 and the numbers start dropping from 2 to 1 to even 0, you can continue. But if you start at the 1 or 2 level and the numbers climb from 3 to 4, you'd better bail out of that workout in a hurry and plan on resting the next few days."

Williams indicates that the pain index can be useful not only during a workout but also 1 or 2 hours afterward, or even the next day. Runners need to determine their discomfort levels before starting to run. If there is any pain, he recommends that they begin by walking, then switch to a jog. If pain continues or gets worse, he has them stop running immediately. "You switch to walking," he advises. "After walking a while, you can try jogging again, but if pain continues, return home immediately."

Runners should record their daily pain index in their training diaries for reference during the rehabilitation phase. "And don't cheat," Williams warns, "because you're only cheating yourself."

Williams offers the scenario on the opposite page as one that typically occurs for runners who become injured.

When icing an injury, Williams suggests using either a commercial ice pack or making your own ice pack by filling a paper cup with water and freezing it. You can then peel off some of the paper to bring the ice in direct contact with the skin. Massage the ice gently across the injured area until the skin turns red and numb. (This should take 5 to 10 minutes.) Then massage for 5 minutes more, but don't overdo the icing.

Williams's Injury Scenario

SYMPTOMS	ACTION
Mild discomfort at end of run	Ice for 10–20 minutes
Some discomfort midrun; does not go away	Take 48 hours off, use an anti-inflammatory drug, cross-train only
Discomfort before going out the door	Run at your own risk, take 72 hours off
Discomfort throughout the day	Don't stall any longer, seek medical help

So that runners do not lose hard-won fitness, Williams recommends that they cross-train during the rehabilitation phase of an injury. Because running is a weight-bearing sport in which the foot contacts the ground on each stride, sending shock waves up the leg, most running injuries are weight-bearing injuries. With this type of injury (such as a twisted ankle), you can't run, or you can't run very fast.

Cross-training permits you to maintain (and sometimes even improve) your base level of fitness by using other sports that either don't stress the injured body part or stress it less than running would. Here, Williams rates some of the sports used in cross-training.

Water training. Swimming and various exercises done in a pool are good, Williams claims, because they stress different muscles than those used in running. "Aquarunning is better than pure swimming because you can more specifically exercise the running muscles," he says. He notes two problems, though: It's more difficult to elevate the heart rate with water exercises because of the pressure of the water, and not everyone has easy access to a swimming pool or a flotation vest. Although runners may start with a vest, Williams suggests that they remove it once they become comfortable in the water. "Treading water provides a much better workout," he says. "You're forced to use your shoulders and arms more. Cupping your hands creates more water drag. Hand flippers make it even tougher." The only negative side to exercising without a vest is that the motions are less specific to motions used in running. But that also can be a positive factor.

Bicycling. This would include riding a stationary bicycle in a gym or an actual bike outdoors. In many respects, indoor cycling is better because of the safety factor. You can't fall off, and you won't be struck by an automobile. Many runners, however, find riding outdoors more interesting. "Even when you start biking, it's easy to raise your heart rate, and most people have a bicycle," Williams says. He believes that fitness enhancement is increased if you include cycling in your training routine each day. You can modulate the level of stress by shifting gears or shifting the lever on an indoor machine.

Exercise machines. The only question here is, Which machines? Cross-country ski simulators have become very popular with people who exercise at home. A newer machine that also exercises both the upper and lower body is the HealthRider. There are dozens of machines on the market that use various levers and pulleys to exercise the upper body. "Not all machines are equal," Williams says. "You have to shop around and find a machine that exercises your body while not aggravating your injury."

Walking. Walking, like running, is a weight-bearing activity, but it places less stress on the lower limbs because the foot doesn't contact the ground so hard. "Walking is an underrated exercise for rehabilitation," Williams says. "Runners don't always like it because they feel they're not accomplishing anything. But you can get a good workout by walking, although you may need to walk longer than you would normally run." Williams cautions again that runners must be symptom-free before beginning to use walking for rehabilitation. If symptoms occur, he has runners wait and rest more before starting up again. (The first stage of his rehabilitation schedule, on the opposite page, uses walking as part of the training mix.)

To this list might be added total rest, which is what you do when your injury prevents you from doing any exercise. Williams cautions about two other activities that, although useful during rehabilitation, have the potential to worsen running injuries.

Stretching. Most knowledgeable runners know the benefits of stretching in promoting flexibility and thereby preventing injuries. But they often stretch more while injured than they would during their regular routine. If they overstretch the injured part of their body, they may actually retard their rehabilitation. "The time to stretch is before you get injured, not after," Williams says. While he considers stretching to be essential to rehabilitative success, he also reminds his runners to warm their muscles before starting to stretch. He believes that one stretch held for 20 seconds or so is not enough to trigger a reflex action, the point where your muscles relax and allow you to extend the stretch. "Forty to 60 seconds works best," he adds. "You have to repeat the stretch three or four times for best results."

Weight lifting. Free weights, particularly, can be a threat to an injured runner because of the danger of extra stress to the legs. "If you have a lower-limb injury," Williams says, "you probably want to avoid lifting weights to strengthen the lower body. But even if you're working on the upper body, you have to pick the weights off the floor, which could cause problems." Because of this, strength machines may be more important during the rehab period. For those without easy access to machines, a rubber tube that can be tied to a doorknob can serve as a handy and inexpensive substitute.

When You're Unable to Walk or Run

During this stage, Williams wants his runners take all of the energy they normally would use to prepare for running competition and channel it into rehabilitation. "The goal is 100 percent recovery," Williams says. "If you only devote 50 percent of your energy to rehabilitation at this point, it is going to delay your return to form that

Week 1					
Day	**Workout**	**Warmup**	**Cross-Training**	**Effort**	**Cooldown**
Mon.	20 min.	3–4 min.	12 min.	Easy	3–4 min.
Tues.	25 min.	3–4 min.	17 min.	Easy	3–4 min.
Wed.	30 min.	3–4 min.	22 min.	Easy	3–4 min.
Thurs.	Rest	—	—	—	—
Fri.	35 min.	3–4 min.	27 min.	Easy	3–4 min.
Sat.	45 min.	3–4 min.	37 min.	Easy	3–4 min.
Sun.	Rest	—	—	—	—

much longer." In addition to the exercises, Williams recommends icing the injury four or five times a day. Stretching is also an important part of this program.

The table on page 193 demonstrates a typical recovery week. The workout is divided into a warmup and cooldown with the cross-training sandwiched between. The level of effort should be easy, about 70 percent of your maximum heart rate. Rest days are as important while cross-training as they are during your regular running training.

Once your body adapts to the cross-training, you can begin training at a harder rate, doing a form of interval training in which you alternate hard and easy efforts in your cross-training exercises. For example, take the workout for Monday and Tuesday below: After warming up at a jog pace, do a half-dozen repeats of 30 seconds at a crisp pace (80 to 84 percent of maximum heart rate), dropping back to a minute or two of easy effort between repeats. Finally, cool down at a jog pace. You can use this same pattern whether you're in a pool, on a bicycle, or using an exercise machine.

Week 2

Day	Workout	Warmup	Cross-Training	Effort	Cooldown
Mon.	25 min.	3–4 min.	6 x 30 sec.	Crisp	3–4 min.
Tues.	25 min.	3–4 min.	6 x 30 sec.	Crisp	3–4 min.
Wed.	35 min.	3–4 min.	6 x 1–2 min.	Hard	3–4 min.
Thurs.	30 min.	3–4 min.	22 min.	Easy	3–4 min.
Fri.	45 min.	3–4 min.	6 x 1–4 min.	Hard	3–4 min.
Sat.	Rest	—	—	—	—
Sun.	60 min.	3–4 min.	52 min.	Easy	3–4 min.

Expect some sore muscles at first if you're not used to the cross-training discipline you choose. If you need more time to adapt, repeat the training pattern above for one or more weeks before shifting to the pattern on the opposite page.

Week 3

Day	Segment 1	Segment 2	Segment 3	Segment 4	Segment 5	Daily Mileage
Mon.	1 mi. walk easy	1 mi. walk medium	0.5 mi. 50/50	—	—	2.5
Tues.	Cross-train	—	—	—	—	—
Wed.	0.5 mi. walk easy	0.5 mi. 50/50	0.5 mi. 150/100	0.5 mi. 250/100	—	2.0
Thurs.	Cross-train	—	—	—	—	—
Fri.	0.5 mi. walk easy	0.5 mi. 50/50	0.5 mi. 150/100	0.5 mi. 250/100	—	2.0
Sat.	Rest	—	—	—	—	—
Sun.	0.5 mi. walk easy	0.5 mi. 50/50	0.5 mi. 100/50	0.5 mi. 250/50	0.5 mi. 100/50	2.5
					Weekly Mileage	9.0

Once you are finished with this cross-training period, hopefully you will be able to return to running. If you are not yet symptom-free, recycle through the program until you can run without pain again.

"You have to be very cautious during rehabilitation," Williams warns, "because if you continue to exercise an injured body part, it delays your full recovery. You must do everything possible to ensure that you will recover as quickly as possible while not reinjuring yourself."

When You're Able to Walk or Jog but Not Run

When runners are symptom-free, Williams has them return to running gradually. "The first day back," Williams says, "I have recovering runners walk 1 mile easy as a warmup. They next walk another mile fairly vigorously. After that, they jog 50 meters, walk 50 meters, jog 50 meters, and so on. This continues for a half-mile. That gives them about 2.5 miles of total activity. We build from that base."

That pattern is reflected in the first Monday workout in the schedule on page 196. "0.5 mi. 50/50" describes the portion of the workout in which the runner covers a half-mile (two laps on the track) alternating 50 meters of jogging and 50 meters of walking. All running should be done at a pace between jog and easy.

Week 4						
DAY	**SEGMENT 1**	**SEGMENT 2**	**SEGMENT 3**	**SEGMENT 4**	**SEGMENT 5**	**DAILY MILEAGE**
MON.	Cross-train	—	—	—	—	—
TUES.	0.5 mi. 50/50	0.5 mi. 100/50	0.5 mi. 200/50	0.5 mi. 400/50	0.5 mi. 200/150	2.5
WED.	Cross-train	—	—	—	—	—
THURS.	0.5 mi. 50/50	0.5 mi. 100/50	0.5 mi . 200/50	1 mi. 400/50	0.5 mi. 200/150	3.0
FRI.	Cross-train	—	—	—	—	—
SAT.	0.5 mi. 100/50	0.5 mi. 400/50	1 mi. 800/50	1 mi. 400/50	—	3.0
SUN.	1 mi. run	5 min. rest	1 mi. run	5 min. rest	1 mi. run	3.0
					WEEKLY MILEAGE	11.5

As in the first phase, if you need more rehabilitative time, simply repeat the last two weeks. If you are able to complete the "test" workout on Sunday of week 4, you are ready to move to the next stage.

When You're Able to Run at an Easy Pace

The final stage, beginning with week 5, blends continuous running at various distances with cross-training of 45 to 60 minutes, both done at an easy pace. At this point, assuming no further injury symptoms develop, you are ready to resume full training.

Final Stage of Rehab							
WEEK	**MON.**	**TUES.**	**WED.**	**THURS.**	**FRI.**	**SAT.**	**SUN.**	**WEEKLY MILEAGE**
5	3 mi. run	Cross-train	4 mi. run	Cross-train	4 mi. run	Cross-train	5–6 mi. run	16–17
6	Cross-train	4 mi. run	Cross-train	5 mi. run	Cross-train	7–8 mi. run	Rest	16–17
7	2 mi. run	4–5 mi. run	2 mi. run	5 mi. run	Cross-train	8 mi. run	Rest	21–22

25

AQUARUNNING
JOE ROGERS'S
WATER-TRAINING PROGRAM

Joe Rogers would prefer to coach running, but like many track coaches these days, he spends a certain amount of time standing on the deck of a swimming pool. "Runners get injured," Rogers admits, "no matter how carefully you try to prepare them. And when they're trying to rehabilitate from injuries, one of the best methods is aquarunning."

Water training (often called aquatraining or aquarunning) is also an efficient method of preventing injuries, suggests Rogers, head coach for men's track and field and cross-country at Ball State University in Muncie, Indiana. By substituting swimming or various activities in the pool that mimic the running motion, runners can gain and maintain fitness while avoiding the pounding that comes from long runs on the roads. "Some athletes are simply more fragile than others," Rogers claims. "If they want to achieve their maximum potential, they need to use alternate methods of training. When I started out in track, we thought the more you ran, the better you got. But that's not necessarily true anymore."

Rogers pole-vaulted for Miami University in Oxford, Ohio, graduating in 1966. Training there at the same time were Bob Schul, 1964 Olympic 5000-meter champion, and Jack Bacheler, who ran in the 1972 Olympic marathon. Rogers coached high school track in Indianapolis, then at Olivet College and Hillsdale College in Michigan before going to Ball State in 1985. His cross-country teams won the Midwest Athletic Conference title in 1987 and qualified for the NCAA championships in 1989. He served as chairman of USA Track and Field's coaching committee between 1993 and 1995 and remains an instructor in that program, which seeks to upgrade the abilities of American track coaches.

"There is no better training for running than running, but overuse injuries, general muscle fatigue, soreness, and boredom are factors that can limit the amount that some individuals can run," Rogers says. He suggests aquarunning as a therapeutic exercise for runners who have reached their mileage limits on the road or track. Here is how Rogers defines some of the forms of water training.

Swimming. Swimming is a fine form of aerobic training for conditioning the cardiovascular system. If you're interested in general fitness, swimming also strengthens the arm and shoulder muscles, which are often overlooked by runners. Although swimming uses different muscles than those used in running, this can be an advantage if those running muscles are injured. Many runners, unfortunately, consider swimming in a pool to be boring.

Kickboard swimming. Swimmers in training often use a kickboard (a foam board that looks like a miniature surfboard). You grasp the board with both hands and use it for buoyancy as you kick with your legs. The advantage of kickboard swimming is that it focuses on many of the same leg muscles used by runners. With certain lower-leg injuries, however, such as those affecting the knees, it may be a good idea to avoid kickboard swimming until the injury begins to heal.

Vest running. Using a flotation vest or other flotation device, runners float in deep water and run in place, mimicking the movements normally used in running. One advantage of this form of aquarunning is that there is little or no stress on the injured body part. A disadvantage is that it is difficult to raise your heart rate. "Running in a vest doesn't offer much resistance," Rogers concedes. He nevertheless considers vest running a good alternative for an athlete who is either injured or on the verge of being overtrained.

Treading water. Many runners who are also good swimmers find that they can shed the vest and obtain a better aerobic workout by simply treading water. The disadvantage is that the arm and leg movements used to stay afloat are less specific to running.

Chest-deep running. Rogers believes that the best form of aquarunning is to move to the shallow end of the pool and run in chest-deep water. "The movements are more specific to running," he says. The water provides enough buoyancy so that the impact forces of the foot contacting the bottom of the pool are limited. For some injured runners, however, any contact may prove impossible.

Water games. Another way to exercise in deep water is to pretend that you are a water polo player and move back and forth across the pool, combining different strokes with treading water and resting. When runners on his track team are doing this type of exercise, Rogers sometimes throws them a water polo ball. "It's a form of play,"

60-Minute Pool Routine

EXERCISE	AREA STRENGTHENED	TIME
Swimming	Arms, shoulders, legs	10 min.
Chest-deep running	Shoulders, hips	15 min.
Kickboard	Legs	5 min.
Vest running	Cardiovascular system	15 min.
Treading water	Arms, shoulders, hips, legs	5 min.
Water games	Total body	10 min.

Rogers suggests. "It offers you one more variation to avoid burnout."

For many runners, a combination of all of the forms of water training may work best together. Rogers suggests the pool routine lasting 60 minutes that is shown on the preceding page.

Once you start training in the water, you may prefer to develop your own training patterns. The nature and degree of your injury also will determine how you train.

Rehabilitation

If and when you become injured, one of the best places to rehabilitate is in a swimming pool. This is particularly true when the injury prohibits you from doing weight-bearing activities. With some injuries, even pedaling an exercise bicycle or using strength machines may be painful. In all rehabilitation, use pain as your guide. "If it hurts, don't do it," Rogers warns.

Concerning the rehabilitative benefits of aquarunning, he explains, "The hydrostatic pressure of water on the limbs massages the injury. Moving the limbs through a full range of motion also helps maintain flexibility during the recovery period. Finally, moving the limbs promotes blood flow to the injured area."

For serious weight-bearing injuries, flotation vests are the first rehabilitative tool to consider. "If the athlete is suspended with a buoyancy vest, he can exercise the lower extremities without any stress," Rogers says.

The rehabilitative training program offered on the opposite page blends the various water training exercises described in the previous section. If any of the activities prove painful, move to a different activity that doesn't stress the injury. The four-week program begins at a base level and progresses by increasing training loads and adding more weight-bearing activities. Four weeks, however, is no magic number. Some runners can spend less time in the pool before returning to running; others may need more time.

In the table, "vest" indicates running in deep water using a flotation vest. On days when multiple exercises are prescribed, light movements while wearing a vest can serve as a warmup and/or cooldown. "Tread" refers to treading water without a vest. "Kick" means to use a kickboard, and "game" means water games. "Inter" refers to a form of interval training while wearing a vest in which you alternate fast movements and slow (recovery) movements, similar to interval training on

Rehabilitation Program

WEEK	MON.	TUES.	WED.	THURS.	FRI.	SAT.	SUN.
1	30 min. vest	10 min. swim 20 min. vest	15 min. vest 5 min. tread 10 min. kick	30 min. vest	10 min. vest 10 min. game 10 min. kick	15 min. swim 15 min. vest	30 min. vest
2	45 min. vest	10 min. vest 5 min. tread 10 min. vest 5 min. tread 10 min. vest	10 min. vest 10 min. chest 10 min. vest 10 min. kick	10 min. vest 15 min. game 10 min. kick 10 min. vest	10 min. vest 30 min. inter 10 min. vest	15 min. swim 15 min. vest	10 min. vest 10 min. chest 10 min. kick 10 min. vest
3	10 min. vest 10 min. tread 10 min. vest 10 min. tread 10 min. vest	15 min. swim 15 min. vest 15 min. kick	10 min. vest 10 min. chest 10 min. vest 10 min. chest 10 min. kick	10 min. vest 15 min. game 10 min. kick 10 min. game 10 min. vest	10 min. vest 20 min. kick	10 min. vest 30–45 min. inter 10 min. vest	15 min. swim 15 min. vest 15 min. kick
4	10 min. vest 30 min. game 10 min. kick	10 min. vest 10 min. chest 10 min. kick 10 min. chest 10 min. kick	10 min. vest 20 min. game 15 min. vest	10 min. vest 5 min. tread 15 min. chest 10 min. kick 15 min. inter	15 min. swim 15 min. vest	10 min. vest 15 min. chest 10 min. kick 15 min. chest 10 min. vest	15 min. vest 15 min. kick 15 min. swim

a track. If your running schedule would have had you running repeats of 5 × 1000, do water repeats for about the same length of time that it would take you to cover that distance running.

As you begin to tolerate weight-bearing activities, which could include walking, jogging, bicycling, or using various exercise machines, you can blend these activities with your aquarunning. Once you're able to run full-time, you might want to consider maintaining some aquarunning as a preventive measure.

Prevention

Many runners have a mileage "red line," which they exceed only at the risk of injury. To avoid future injuries, substitute aquarunning for some of your running. Or you can use it to increase your total training time without increasing mileage and the pounding you get on the road. Water training also can be used as a substitute exercise when weather (hot or cold) makes running outdoors uncomfortable.

The four-week training program below is designed for an intermediate runner who is already in good physical condition and is preparing for a 5-K race. It substitutes two to three water workouts a week for running workouts. Use the 60-minute routine described on page 198 or any of the workouts in the rehabilitation program. Although this table is specific to a certain skill level, you can use the pattern to adapt any training program to include aquarunning.

Run/Swim Program

WEEK	MON.	TUES.	WED.	THURS.	FRI.	SAT.	SUN.
1	30 min. jog	8 x 400 crisp	60 min. pool	5 x 1000 medium	45 min. pool	Tempo run	60 min. easy
2	30 min. pool	12 x 200 hard	60 min. pool	3 x 1 mi. medium	45 min. pool	Fartlek	75 min. easy
3	30 min. jog	8 x 400 crisp	60 min. pool	5 x 1000 medium	45 min. pool	Tempo run	90 min. easy
4	30 min. pool	12 x 200 hard	30 min. pool	3 x 1 mi. medium	Rest	**5–K RACE**	60 min. easy

26

WEIGHT LOSS
JUDY TILLAPAUGH'S
FAT-BURNING PROGRAM

It is the contention of Judy Tillapaugh, R.D., that while many experts who instruct people on how to lose weight state that the only successful regimen is one that combines diet and exercise, few tell you exactly how to do it. "The unanswered questions are how much to eat," Tillapaugh says, "and how much to exercise."

Tillapaugh herself has done a good job of combining a healthy eating regimen with exercise. She began running in eighth grade in Ithaca, New York. She ran track and cross-country at Purdue University in Indiana, qualifying for the NCAA Championships in 1979 with a time of 36:42 for 10,000 meters. After graduation in 1982, she went to work as a dietitian at St. Joseph's Medical Center in Fort Wayne, Indiana, and became active in the Fort Wayne Track Club and the Road Runners Club of America (RRCA). She served as president of the Fort Wayne club, rose to regional director of the RRCA, and still found time to run a 3:04 marathon. In the fall of 1995, Tillapaugh became women's cross-country and track coach at Indiana University–Purdue University at Fort Wayne, where she also acts as wellness and fitness coordinator.

As a registered dietitian, Tillapaugh frequently counsels runners on their nutritional needs. "Losing weight is simple—in theory," she says. "If you burn more calories than you consume, you'll lose weight. It's calories in versus calories out. But in practice, it doesn't always work that smoothly."

Although the numbers may vary somewhat from individual to individual, depending on size, if you consume an extra 3,500 calories, you'll gain 1 pound. If you burn an extra 3,500 calories from exercise, you'll lose 1 pound. A can of nondiet soda contains 150 calories. Drink a case of soda, and (after normal fluid loss) you'll be 1 pound heavier. Run or walk 1 mile, and you'll burn approximately 100 calories, so it takes 36 of those miles to balance the calorie gain from the 24 cans of soda.

The most effective way to lose weight is to combine exercise with a healthy eating plan in order to create a daily calorie deficit. If you usually eat 2,000 calories a day and you go on a 1,500-calorie diet— and everything else is equal—you can lose a pound a week. The arithmetic is fairly simple: 7 × 500 calories less per day = 3,500 calories = 1 pound lost. Or you can increase your calorie expenditure by exercising. Running 5 miles a day will have the same effect; the arithmetic is the same. Or you can eat 1,800 calories a day (a 200-calorie deficit) and run 3 miles a day (300 calories burned). The result is the same: A 500-calorie deficit and a guaranteed weight loss if pursued over a period of time.

That sounds easy, but if you're running for fitness or training for competition, you need a well-balanced diet and enough calories to provide the energy you need to exercise. Starvation diets don't work and will make you a less effective runner. Tillapaugh considers 1 pound a week a healthy weight loss. "It's nearly impossible to shed fat fast," she warns. Quick-weight-loss programs succeed partly because of fluid loss, which is temporary. "People have a higher chance of success if they follow a realistic and healthy weight-loss plan, which also permits them to gain fitness," Tillapaugh says. She recommends that people eat foods they like and choose exercises they enjoy.

"People first need to determine their calorie needs, how much they need for weight gain or weight loss. After that, they need a nutrition plan that they can combine with an exercise plan." Tillapaugh believes that 1,500 calories a day is a safe and realistic goal for most women if they want to lose weight, especially if they are active in running or walking. Men generally have more muscle mass and burn more calories than women, so an active man who is somewhat larger might succeed on 1,800 to 2,000 calories a day.

Dietitians use different formulas to determine calorie needs. One developed by Harris Benedict in 1919 is still in use. The Benedict formula for determining basic energy expenditure for women is 665 + (9.6 × kilograms of body weight) + (1.7 × centimeters of height) −(4.7 × age).

As if this isn't complicated enough, the Benedict formula for determining basic energy expenditure for men is slightly different: 66 + (13.7 × kilograms of body weight) + (5 × centimeters of height) − (6.8 × age).

To use the formula, you first need to convert to the metric system: To get the metric numbers, divide your weight in pounds by 2.2 and multiply your height in inches by 2.54.

As for the rationale behind the strange numbers above, don't even ask. But dietitians find the formula handy in designing eating plans for their clients. And you may find it similarly useful if you want to compute your eating needs.

The Benedict formula, however, only allows you to estimate how many calories you would burn if you remained inactive and didn't get out of bed each day. Simply by moving around, you will burn additional calories. Sitting in front of a computer burns calories. Chewing food burns calories, although nowhere near as many as you consume while eating that food.

The point is that once you determine your basic energy expenditure, you need to factor in your normal activity level (usually 30 to 40 percent of the basic number). If you exercise, you will have to do additional calculations based on the amount and type of exercise you do.

As an example, the tables on the opposite page show the numbers for a woman runner who is 5 feet 6 inches tall (167.64 centimeters), weighs 150 pounds (68.18 kilograms), and is 35 years old.

The Benedict formula allows us to estimate how many calories this runner burns daily: $665 + (9.6 \times 68.18$ kilograms$) + (1.7 \times 167.64$ centimeters$) - (4.7 \times 35$ years$) = 1,440.02$ calories.

Don't put the calculator away yet—you're not finished. That is merely the number of calories the sample runner would burn daily if she never stirred out of bed. During her regular daily activities, she would burn more calories, which would be her normal activity level. Assuming that to be 30 percent of the number above, her normal activity level would be $1,440.02 \times 0.30 = 432$.

To that you must add the exercise level. If the sample athlete runs 3 miles a day, at 100 calories per mile, she burns 300 additional calories.

Getting there has been somewhat complicated, but you now can calculate the runner's caloric expenditure (and energy needs) for a day on which she ran 3 miles. Her basic energy expenditure (1,440.02) plus her normal activity level (432) equals her total basic expenditure (1,872.02). Add to that her exercise level (300), and you come up with her total caloric expenditure for the day (2,172.02).

The number to pay attention to is the approximately 1,870 calories that she burns each day with *no* exercise. If she eats more than that number of calories, she will gain weight. If she eats less, she will lose weight. Running 3 miles increases her total calories burned to 2,170, allowing her to lose weight faster or maintain it with more calories in her diet. Let's see how it works using a menu that provides 1,500 calories a day.

Not everybody follows the same activity pattern day after day. On Tuesday, our average runner does no running, although she follows the same 1,500-calorie eating plan.

A week's eating and running would result in the calorie balances shown on page 208.

Monday

CALORIES CONSUMED		CALORIES BURNED	
BREAKFAST	Cereal w/banana 1 cup skim milk	Basic energy expenditure	1,440
LUNCH	Turkey sandwich w/mustard 1 tomato 1 apple	Normal activity level	432
DINNER	3 oz. lean beef Baked potato w/margarine Carrots Salad w/dressing 1 cup skim milk	Subtotal	1,872
SNACKS	3 cups popcorn 1/2 cup orange juice	Exercise level (3-mi. run)	300
TOTAL CALORIES	1,500	**TOTAL CALORIES**	2,172
		CALORIE BALANCE	−672

Tuesday

CALORIES CONSUMED		CALORIES BURNED	
BREAKFAST	1 cup oatmeal w/cinnamon 1 sliced apple 1/2 cup orange juice 1 cup skim milk	Basic energy expenditure	1,440
LUNCH	1 tuna pita 1 pear 1 cup V-8	Normal activity level	432
DINNER	3 oz. pork chop Mashed potatoes Green beans 1 roll w/margarine 1 cup skim milk	Subtotal	1,872
SNACKS	Fruit and pretzels Water	Rest	0
TOTAL CALORIES	1,500	**TOTAL CALORIES**	1,872
		CALORIE BALANCE	−372

A Week's Worth of Calorie Balances

DAY	MILES	EXERCISE CALORIES	BASE CALORIES EXPENDED	TOTAL CALORIES	CALORIES CONSUMED	CALORIE BALANCE
MON.	3	300	1,872	2,172	1,500	−672
TUES.	5	500	1,872	2,372	1,500	−872
WED.	0	0	1,872	1,872	1,500	−372
THURS.	3	300	1,872	2,172	1,500	−672
FRI.	5	500	1,872	2,372	1,500	−872
SAT.	3	300	1,872	2,172	1,500	−672
SUN.	0	0	1,872	1,872	1,500	−372
				CALORIE BALANCE FOR WEEK		−4,504

Since 1 pound equals 3,500 calories, that much exercise in a week coupled with a daily 1,500-calorie diet would result in the loss of more than a pound a week. In fact, with nearly 1,000 calories to spare, you could treat yourself to a piece of pie or an ice cream cone, confident that you will still lose 1 pound.

The schedules in this chapter should be considered only as guidelines, not specifics that you can follow precisely. (For a more precise nutrition plan, you might want to consider consulting a registered dietitian, who can cater to your likes and dislikes when it comes to eating.) Men and women do differ. Diets vary. Training levels may change. Nevertheless, the same principles apply. If you burn more calories than you consume, you will lose weight. If the opposite is true, the pounds will continue to accumulate. Once you achieve your desired weight, you can maintain it by adding back calories to match your weight-maintenance needs.

INDEX

Hard pace, 13
Hard/easy pace, 13
Hardening, for ultramarathon, 87
Hayes, Dean, 26
Headwear, in hot weather, 148
Heart monitor, 13
Heart rates, maximum, 5–8
Heatstroke, 146
Hills, 143
    repeats in training for, 33
    track phase for, 114–15
    training for, 13–14
Hoag, Steve, 137
Hodgkinson, Toni, 111–12
Holmer, Gosta, 13
Hormone replacement therapy, women
        runners and, 130
Hydration, 147

I

Injury
    preventing, 202
    scenario for repairing, 191
Interval training, 14, 32
Ironman Triathlon, 172

J

Joe Rogers's Water-Training Program,
        197–202
Jog pace, 14
Jog/walk pace, 38
John Davies's Phased Program, 110–19
Johnson, Tom, 86, 90
Jones, Kim, 66
Judy Tillapaugh's Fat-Burning Program, 203–8

K

Kapkori, Joseph, 103–4
Kennedy, Bob, 101, 103
Klecker, Barney
    Boston Marathon program, 142–45
    cold weather training, 136–45

L

Lactic acid, 14
Lange, Hank, triathlon program, 171–77
LaSalle Banks Chicago Marathon, 1
Legs, exercises for, 182
Long runs, 14, 67–68
Long walks, 165
Lunges, 184

Lydiard, Arthur, 13, 110
Lydiardism, 111

M

Marathon, viii–ix, 55
Marathoners
    expert schedules, 63–65
    intermediate schedules, 60–63
    novice schedules, 58–60
Marathon(s), 14
    Benji Durden's elite program, 66–76
    Boston, 17, 142–45
    Brian Piper's Chicago program for, 54–65
    Chicago, viii, 54–65
    City of Lakes, 137
    cold weather training for, 142–45
    cross-training for, 79
    Dallas White Rock, 57
    Disney World, 147
    focusing on goal for, 56–58
    Grandma's, 57, 136, 138
    half-, 44–47
    hot weather training for, 153
    LaSalle Banks, 1
    Marine Corps, 77–84, 147
    Memphis, 78, 84
    multiple, 77–84
    Napa Valley, 147
    National Capital, 129
    Olympic Trials, 137
    runner levels in, 56, 58–65
    time in, 56–57
    training programs between multiple, 81–83
    Twin Cities, 57, 137
    ultra, 18, 85–91
    Vulcan, 146–47
Marine Corps Marathon, 77–84, 147
Mark Fenton's Fitness Walking Program,
        155–61
Martin Rudow's 30-Week Peak Program,
        162–70
Massage, 15
Masters, 15
Max, 15
Maximum heart rates (MHR), 5, 15
Maximum training, 68
Medicine ball, in strength training, 181, 183
Medium pace, 15
Memphis Marathon, 78, 84
Menstruation, 130–31
Meters, 15–16

Roy Benson's Speed-Improvement Program, 31–36
RRCA, 203
Rudow, Martin
   Advanced Race Walking, 162
   set workouts, 166
   30-week program, 162–70
Run Fast, viii–ix
Runner's World, vii–viii, 2, 14, 55
   "The Path to Marathon Success," 66
Running terms, 10–19
Running Trax, 16
Run/Swim Program, 202

S

Salt, in hot weather, 147–48
Sam Bell's Training Program, 101–9
Saucony Triathlon, 172
Savage, Paddy, first-timers' program, 25–30
Semi-stress workouts, 102
Step-ups, 184
Shamrock Marathon, 77–84
Sheehan, George, 14
Sit-ups, 182
Skiing, cross-country, 139–40
Skill level, for Boston Marathon, 142
Snell, Peter, 110
Snowshoeing, 139
Speed
   drills for triathlon, 175
   vs. endurance, 179
   training, 32–33, 68
      base phases, 33–36
   in walking, 160–61
Speedwork, 17, 32, 143, 149
   summer, 151
Spivey, Jim, 101
Splits, 17
Sprint pace, 17
Squats, 184
Squires, Bill, 48
Stazinski, Rich, 3
   training paces of, 4
Strength
   building, 185–87
   training, 17–18, 140–41, 178–87
   for triathlon, 175–76
Stress
   measuring, 7
   test, 18
Stress workouts, 102

Stretching, 18, 192–93
   for triathlon, 175–76
Stride(s), 18, 164
Strolling, 165
Summer. *See also* Weather
   cross-country training, 106–7
   early training, 103–4
   girls' cross-country in, 93–94
Sunburn, preventing, 148
Surges, 10, 18
Swimming, 198–99
   in triathalon, 173
Switzer, Kathrine, 17

T

Taper, 18
   in strength training, 187
Taylor, Mary, 94
Tempo run, 18, 69
   in summer, 151–52
Tempo walks, 165
10-K
   basic training program, 37–43
   children's, 121–22
   eight-week training schedule for, 38–40
   improving times, 40–42
Tillapaugh, Judy, fat-burning program, 203–8
Track, phased program for, 110–19
Track-and-field coaching, 179
Training effect, 18
Training paces
   Bell's, 3
   Benson's, 6
   Stazinski's, 4
Treading water, 199
Triathlon(s)
   bicycling in, 173
   buildup for, 174–76
   double sports in, 175
   Hank Lange's program, 171–77
   Ironman, 172
   pickups for, 175
   running in, 173
   Saucony, 172
   six-week phase schedule for, 176
   speed drills for, 175
   strength and stretching for, 175–76
   swimming in, 173
   transition during, 173–74
   tuneup for, 176–77